# Classroom evaluation strategies

# Classroom evaluation strategies

**ELIZABETH C. KING, Ph.D.**

Assistant Professor,
Department of Health Education Professions,
State University of New York,
Buffalo, New York

with 27 illustrations

**The C. V. Mosby Company**

ST. LOUIS • TORONTO • LONDON    1979

Printed in the United States of America

The C. V. Mosby Company
11830 Westline Industrial Drive, St. Louis, Missouri 63141


**Library of Congress Cataloging in Publication Data**

King, Elizabeth C             1941-
    Classroom evaluation strategies.

    Bibliography: p.
    Includes index.
    1.   Nursing—Study and teaching.   2.   Educational tests and measurements.   3.   Nursing—Examinations.
I.   Title.
RT73.K56             .610.73'076            79-13907
ISBN 0-8016-2674-9


C/M/M  9  8  7  6  5  4  3  2  1     01/D/067

*In memoriam*

**ANTHONY J. CAMP**

(1911-1972)

# Preface

This book has been written primarily for nursing educators and prospective nursing educators who are daily responsible for planning and evaluating instruction. The systematic approach to instructional design provides the basic conceptual framework for the text. The text does not contain all that the educator should know about the evaluation of instruction; rather, it focuses on the evaluation of classroom learning. It is designed to provide the instructor with a basic strategy for integrating evaluation into overall instructional planning and design.

General guidelines for constructing objective and essay tests are discussed, and relevant nursing examples are given. The concepts of test validity and reliability as they relate to both teacher-made and standardized tests are presented. Common statistical indices are discussed. An understanding of these statistical techniques will help the instructor interpret test scores. Although assessing human behavior and performance is hazardous and subject to error, a well-designed test with a carefully interpreted score is preferable to subjective data. A small portion of the text is devoted to motivation and test anxiety. Finally, the book ends with a discussion of grading and some of the dilemmas faced by all of us as we try to quantify data that are both objective and subjective into some meaningful symbol.

My hope for all instructors using this text is that they not misuse their test scores but place test scores into proper perspective, weighing scores as only one source of data for decision making and remembering that not everyone will learn the same thing, the same way, at the same rate.

As educators, we must be ever conscious of our impact on our students' self-image. When evaluating, we need to separate the test score from the person. Our students must know that we believe they can fail a test but not be a failure, that we are open to other viewpoints, that we see the gray in a seemingly only black and white issue.

We can neither make our students learn nor learn for them; we can only provide the setting and experiences for learning.

I would like to express my appreciation to those who assisted in the development of this book. Thank you: to the writers whose ideas are acknowledged in this text; to Dolores Filson, the editor; to Monica Stenson, for typing the final copy, preparing the illustrations, and typing revisions for the chapter on statistics; to H. Irene Johnson and Arlene D. Batt for helping Monica type early drafts; and to Paul, Thomas, and John for sharing in my pleasure on completion of the text.

**Elizabeth C. King**

# Contents

**1 Systematic instructional design, 1**

Rationale, 2
Goals and objectives, 3
Preassessment, 5
Learning strategies, 7
Postassessment, 23
Instructional revision, 24

**2 Constructing classroom achievement tests, 27**

Defining objectives, 27
Constructing a table of specifications, 28
Writing test directions, 33
Writing test items, 34
Summary, 42

**3 The essay question, 44**

Designing essay test items, 46
Guidelines for writing essay test items, 51
Types of essay test items, 53
Guidelines for grading essay test items, 54
Summary, 56

**4 Basic test attributes, 58**

Validity, 58
Reliability, 66
Practicality, 71
Summary, 72

**5 A few statistics, 74**

Frequency distributions: organization and presentation of data, 74
Descriptive statistics, 83
Summary, 122

ix

6  **Item analysis,** 125

Purposes of item analysis, 125
Interpreting item analysis indices, 126
Manual item analysis, 129
Computer output for item analysis, 131
Test item file, 133
Limitations of item analysis for teacher-made tests, 135
Item analysis for criterion-referenced tests, 135
Summary, 139

7  **Psychosocial concerns for testing,** 140

Behaviorist approach, 140
Test anxiety, 147
Summary, 150

8  **Grading,** 152

Norm-referenced grades, 152
Criterion-referenced grades, 156
Noneducational causes of academic failure, 165
Growth versus achievement, 166
Weighing assessment data, 167
Grade inflation, 168
Summary, 169

# Classroom evaluation strategies

# 1

# Systematic instructional design

The systems approach to instruction is not, as some of the uninitiated assume, a cold, mechanical process. It does not restrict or dictate curriculum or course content. Rather, it is a conceptual framework easily applied to any course content.

The systems approach is especially well suited to nursing instruction because it encompasses not only the teaching of facts and principles but also the development of attitudes and values and it permits an unlimited variety of teaching/learning situations. This chapter presents the systems approach to teaching/learning and illustrates how nursing faculty can use this approach to monitor the quality of their instruction.

Instructional systems models have found increasingly broad application and acceptance in education generally (Popham and Baker, 1970, Roueche and Pitman, 1972) and in medical and health-related curricula in particular (Heidgerken, 1965, Holcomb and Garner, 1973, Segall and others, 1975).

There are several reasons for using a systematic approach to instruction. Some of these are:
- To provide a more integrated, coordinated, and complete program of instruction.
- To provide for consideration of individual differences, for example, in academic background, learning style, and previous clinical experience.
- To provide competency-based instruction.
- To ensure a systematic development of learning experiences through the use of appropriate teaching methods and materials.
- To establish a reliable and valid means of assessment.

As nursing educators use the systems approach to instruction to design learning experiences, they realize the benefit of integrated planning. The following advantages also become evident:
- The applicability of systematized approaches for both undergraduate and graduate nursing programs.

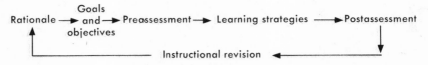

Fig. 1-1. A systems model for instruction.

- The desirability of changing from teaching-oriented to learning-oriented modes of instruction.
- The variety of methods, materials, and assessment procedures available to expand and reinforce instruction.
- The way in which a competency-based format of instruction contributes to a nonthreatening learning and testing environment.
- The ease of identifying and measuring changes in the student's behavior after instruction and of documenting those changes to produce a strong statement of instructional accountability.

Many systems models have been developed and are useful for instructional planning. The model presented here has been discussed extensively by Roueche and Pitman (1972) and includes as the system's components rationale, goals and objectives, preassessment, learning strategies, postassessment, and instructional revision. The system is represented in Fig. 1-1.

All of the elements of the model are interactive, each representing a specific task; they build on one another to create the desired change in behavior. The instructional revision component interacts throughout in a cyclical feedback process to monitor all phases of the system continuously. Other models are more complex and sophisticated, with more components and variables involved in instructional planning. However, although Fig. 1-1 represents a simplistic system, it is not simple. It works as well as other, more complex models and provides the instructional planner with a basic conceptual framework that may be applied to a variety of instructional problems.

The remainder of this chapter presents each component of the competency-based model as it relates to instructional planning for nursing educators.

## RATIONALE

A rationale statement provides the student with some explanation or justification for studying a unit. A written rationale statement provides the instructor the opportunity to explain and justify selecting the content included in a particular unit of study. A rationale statement helps answer content questions students may ask: "Why take statistics? My primary goal is pediatric nursing." "Of what practical value is memorizing the Krebs cycle?" "Why should I learn about the history of psychotherapy? I only want to know what's happening with mental illness today!"

These are not cynical questions revealing rejection of traditional nursing instruction. Rather, they are examples of student concern for relevant, significant course content. Student demands for rationale statements are valid. While pointing out important course or unit content, rationale statements also provide students with a sense of self-direction and purpose. For example, a rationale statement for a unit on community mental health programs may be written as follows:

> Although enduring cures for mental disorders have been elusive, psychoactive drugs together with community treatment programs have markedly reduced the number of people in mental hospitals. The focus of care has shifted from isolated wards within state hospitals to community facilities. Whatever its future evolution, psychotherapy with the use of psychoactive drugs has forever changed the treatment of mental illness. An in-depth study of community mental health programs will be the primary focus of this learning unit.

## GOALS AND OBJECTIVES

The first step in the identification of goals is to specify the competencies or tasks an entry-level nurse must exhibit. The essential question to be asked is: What are the necessary competencies for the entry-level nurse? The competencies identified should encompass all the tasks and responsibilities necessary for the entry-level practitioner. These competencies can be developed and validated by on-the-job task analysis and the use of advisory committees. Once overall program goals are identified, specific competency-based objectives may be developed.

A goal is a broad statement of purpose. It should represent a logical implementation of a well-defined need. Goals are not written in terms of precise, observable behavior. Instead, they are broad statements describing overall learning outcomes in nonspecific terms.

Sample goal statements are:

- The student will assist the patient with activities of daily living and encourage appropriate self-care.
- The student will administer medications and therapeutic treatments prescribed for the patient.
- The student will be able to recognize stresses in human relationships between patients, patients' families, visitors, and health care personnel.

Notice that the goals are in the form of general statements and are not always expressed in terms of measurable, observable behavior. Instead, they describe overall learning outcomes. They provide an overall description of the learning experience. Competency-based instruction accepts goal setting as the prerequisite to effective teaching and evaluation.

In contrast to goals, competency-based objectives are more specific statements that describe observable student behavior. The key to writing competency-based objectives is to develop a basic honesty about what is required and what is not (Roueche, 1976). When instructors clearly define what they hope to accomplish, both students and instructors experience minimal frustration when evaluation of performance is accomplished.

Having selected specific goals for a nursing program, instructors can identify specific competency-based objectives. Competency-based objectives are a type of behavioral objective. Their most important feature is their evolution from the overall goals previously identified.

Competency-based objectives can be established by asking the following question: When a nurse exhibits a specific competency, what is the underlying cognitive, psychomotor, and/or affective base for that specific competency? The answer can be stated in terms of specific behaviors that the student should be able to exhibit. These behaviors can then be classified and sequenced.

The answer also assumes a knowledge of the taxonomy, or classification, of behavioral objectives in three domains of learning: the cognitive domain, the psychomotor domain, and the affective domain.

1. Cognitive objectives focus on what the student is to know. An objective in the cognitive domain requires the student to recall, comprehend, apply, synthesize, analyze, and/or evaluate knowledge.
2. Psychomotor, or performance, objectives are primarily concerned with behavioral tasks involving muscular action or control. An objective in the psychomotor domain requires the student to perform skill procedures encompassing perceptual motor tasks.
3. Affective objectives are concerned with beliefs, attitudes, values, and perceptions. An objective in the affective domain requires the student to internalize a value or belief.

Further classification of objectives has been documented by Mager (1962), Cohen (1974), Bloom (1956), Krathwohl, Bloom, and Masia (1964), and Simpson (1972). Since the focus of this passage is primarily the identification and evaluation of cognitive learning objectives, in-depth exploration of these classifications is not conducted here.

A well-written competency-based objective includes the following (Mager, 1962):

- Description of what the student is to do.
- Outline of conditions under which the student will do it.
- Specification of the level of achievement the student should attain.

For example, specific competency-based objectives relative to the overall goals presented previously might be:

- The student will be able to list the six food groups involved in the diabetic exchange pattern and their respective values with 100% accuracy.
- The student will be able to instruct the patient to independently administer insulin so that, when the patient is discharged, he or she can independently administer insulin.
- The student will be able to counsel the stroke patient's family so they can participate in the patient's rehabilitation.

Critics of behavioral objectives argue that actions which can be stated in behavioral terms tend not to be very important, that behaviorally stated objectives limit achievement by putting ceilings on student aspirations, and that it is impossible to specify and evaluate all the outcomes that might be accomplished by instruction (Trimble, 1973).

Advocates of behavioral objectives counter these arguments with: Important or not, you can never measure intangibles; thus it is far better to concentrate on the attainable. Second, attainment of objectives does not diminish student aspirations but motivates students. However, the third criticism, that it is impossible to evaluate all instructional outcomes, is probably applicable. We can probably never measure the total impact of the nursing curriculum on our students. This criticism does not diminish the importance of defining with clarity what we are trying to accomplish.

Although behaviorally stated objectives are not the panacea for curing all the ills of education, they are an attempt to facilitate honest, effective communication between the nursing instructor and the student. They provide a direction for learning and specify evaluation criteria.

## PREASSESSMENT

Students' prior learning always affects the way they achieve new learning. Consequently, to develop the most effective teaching/

ASSUME ALL KNOW                 PREASSESS                 OBJECTIVE

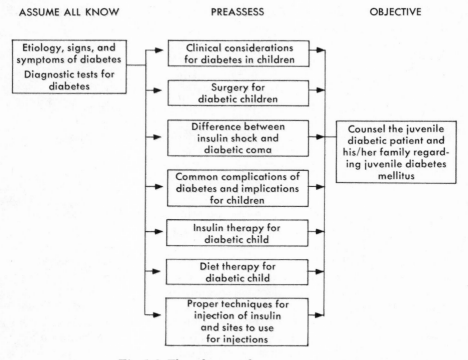

**Fig. 1-2.** Flow diagram for preassessment.

learning sequences, the instructor must determine what knowledge and skills the nursing student brings to the classroom or clinical setting. Instruction simply cannot accommodate differences if it cannot distinguish the differences.

Preassessment is a check on the current status of the student's knowledge and skill in reference to a planned future status. In practice, preassessment is often merely a verbal check, and at times this may be sufficient. However, nothing can take the place of thorough knowledge of the student's abilities before instruction begins.

The best way to determine if students can perform a psychomotor task is to have them actually perform it. In contrast, to preassess cognitive information, a written pretest is recommended. The written pretest may be the course or unit final examination. Obviously, some assumptions regarding previous learning must be made or preassessment becomes too cumbersome to be practical.

Fig. 1-2 provides an example of planning for preassessment (Wong and Raulerson, 1974).

In order to conduct preassessment, the instructor must understand what skills the student will need in order to accomplish the objective. Thus, an analysis of the learning tasks necessary is required. For example, the objective and the learning tasks necessary to meet the objective presented in Fig. 1-2 could be stated in the following manner:

**Learning tasks**

**1.10** Affective skills necessary

    1.11 Demonstrate the interaction skill of expressing empathy

    1.12 Demonstrate the interaction skill of showing positive regard

    1.13 Apply the interaction skill of reducing threat

    1.14 Be aware of the need to develop trust

**1.20** Communication skills necessary

    1.21 Demonstrate attending behavior techniques

    1.22 Demonstrate paraphrasing techniques

    1.23 Illustrate the use of reflection of feeling

    1.24 Develop the ability to summarize content

Now that an analysis of the learning tasks necessary to accomplish the course objective and a preassessment have been conducted, the instructor can begin to develop appropriate learning strategies.

## LEARNING STRATEGIES

Planning for the presentation of content requires integration of the decisions about the selection of appropriate *teaching methods* and those about the selection of appropriate *media*.

## Methods

There are at least four guidelines one may consider when determining appropriate teaching methods.

1. *The teaching method must be suited to the objectives and the content characteristics.* Depending on the objectives to be met, certain instructional methods may be superior. Davies (1973) has summarized the relevant research literature and suggests the following generalizations in choosing an appropriate teaching method:

- All teaching strategies can be used to accomplish "cognitive" objectives. However, lower-order cognitive objectives can best be accomplished by lecture, lecture-discussion, programmed instruction, and computer-assisted instruction, whereas higher-order cognitive objectives can be accomplished by all teaching strategies.
- Lower-order "affective" objectives (those emphasizing receiv-

ing, responding, valuing) can be effectively taught by utilizing all teaching strategies. Higher-order affective objectives (those emphasizing organizing and internalizing) can be most effectively taught by group discussion, role playing, case studies, leaderless groups, and sensitivity training.

- "Psychomotor" objectives are best accomplished by lecture-demonstration, practical tutorials, and independent study with practice.

2. *The instructor must have knowledge of learning and motivational theory before choosing a particular teaching method.* The following principles of learning and motivation are brief statements derived from the writings of learning theorists. These principles should be considered before selection of a teaching method.

- *Students are likely to be motivated to learn things that are meaningful* (Ausubel, 1968). Ausubel argues that new material must relate to information already acquired by the student. When new material is related to previously acquired knowledge, the new information is more easily acquired and remembered.

- *Students are more likely to learn something new if they have all the prerequisites* (Ausubel, 1968, Gagne, 1970). Ausubel emphasizes the necessity of previous knowledge being mastered before new information is given. Furthermore, Ausubel suggests that the weak predictive validity of some pretests is a direct result of the inadequate estimate of the student's prior cognitive knowledge. Similarly, Gagne recommends that before teaching new tasks, the instructor should ensure that all prerequisite tasks have been mastered.

- *Students are more likely to acquire new behavior if they are presented with a model performance to watch and imitate* (Bandura and Walters, 1963). Perhaps the greatest advantage of learning by imitation is that it provides a complete behavioral sequence for the learner.

- *Students are more likely to learn by novel presentations* (Ausubel, 1968). In Ausubel's system, the ability to remember is a function of whether or not the new material can be disassociated from existing material. Consequently, if new material is very similar to existing material, it will be forgotten more quickly; if new material is an extension of existing material but novel, it will be remembered for a longer period of time.

- *Students are more likely to learn if instructional conditions are made pleasant* (Skinner, 1969). Skinner argues that much of current educational practice is based on aversive control. This aversive control is used for both disciplinary and instructional purposes. He recommends positive reinforcement of desired behavior and ignoring of undesirable behavior as the means to produce a more warm and rewarding classroom environment.

- *Students are more likely to learn if they are actively involved in the instructional process.* Active involvement in the learning process is more effective than mere observation. The opportunity to actively apply new knowledge is essential to learning success and increased retention. Active involvement in the learning process is critical to the development of psychomotor skills.
- *The teaching/learning experience must provide the necessary conditions for the transfer of knowledge* (Bruner, 1966). Bruner encourages instructors to develop exercises and learning conditions that will facilitate the student's discovering the conceptual linkage between events. This conceptual linkage will maximize the possibility of the transfer of learning.

3. *The instructor should consider the learning style preferences of students when choosing an appropriate teaching method.* The Canfield-Lafferty Learning Styles Inventory yields data that can be useful to the nursing instructor (Canfield and Lafferty, 1974). Instructors can determine their preferred learning styles and use this information to avoid imposing their preferences on students. More important, the Learning Styles Inventory can be used to determine learning style preferences of individual students and groups of students. With learning styles information, the teacher can develop a variety of classroom and clinical experiences to reach the maximum number of students.

It has been suggested that Learning Styles Inventory results be used to match students and teachers. However, with the limited supply of nursing educators, this is an unrealistic suggestion. It is possible that our educational environment might be enriched by these differences.

4. *The teaching method should be efficient.* For example, the use of small-group seminars to disseminate knowledge may be preferred by some students, but it is obviously not as efficient as the lecture method. Clinical education is very expensive in terms of time, supplies, and personnel involved. However, it is a critical component of any nursing program because of the higher-level learning involved, including the application, analysis, synthesis, and evaluation of knowledge; the demonstration and practice of psychomotor skills; and the demonstration and practice of affective learning appropriate for the clinical setting.

Any adequate discussion of the systems approach must consider teaching methods. Eight teaching methods are presented and discussed briefly: lecture, lecture-discussion, group discussion, role playing, demonstration, laboratory method, independent study, and individualized instruction (namely, autotutorial instruction, programmed instruction and computer-assisted instruction). Learning and reviewing teaching methods comprise one way for the instructor to revitalize the classroom.

### Lecture

The lecture is still the most widely used method for the transmittal of knowledge in the classroom. It is currently being severely criticized as a teaching method because of its long history of misuse or overuse. It is misused when other teaching methods are recommended for achieving the learning objectives.

The advantages of the lecture method are the following:
- Lectures can help clarify ideas and concepts by the incorporation of concrete illustrations, explanatory models, and explanations of how concepts learned can transfer to other situations.
- Lectures can bring facts and ideas alive from the printed page.
- Lecures can expose many students to living authorities.
- Lectures can allow the nursing instructor's enthusiasm, experience, and expertise in organizing knowledge to motivate students and clarify reading material.

In contrast, one of the major criticisms of the lecture method is that the learner is passive. This passivity may result in withdrawal if the learner becomes confused. Often the learner may become so busy taking notes that there is little time to integrate the information being presented.

The lecture method is most suitable (Mizell and Bell, 1977):
- When practitioners agree on the major concepts, principles, and skills.
- For conveying knowledge and organizing material.
- For motivating students and arousing interest in a subject.
- When the material must be remembered for only a short time.
- When it is necessary to provide an introduction to a new topic or concept, explain a process, or provide directions for learning tasks to be implemented by another method.

In contrast, Mizell and Bell (1977) argue that lectures are not appropriate when:
- Long-term retention is necessary.
- The material is complex, detailed, or abstract.

- Learner participation is necessary to the achievement of the course objectives.
- Higher-level cognitive objectives (analysis, synthesis, or evaluation) must be attained.

However, since the lecture method is so widely used, constant efforts should be made to adequately prepare faculty to use the method.

### Lecture-discussion

The lecture-discussion is another teaching strategy used frequently by nursing instructors. The lecture portion is often enhanced by audiovisual aids, and students are encouraged to interrupt for questions, comments, and clarification. It can effectively be used to explain concepts and principles. The discussion portion can provide students the opportunity to explore relationships and develop generalizations. By actively participating in the discussion, students begin to develop skill in critical thinking.

Teaching skills are defined as the set of instructional techniques that make up the teaching process. They can be used singly or collectively to improve the instructor's skill at lecture-discussion. Microteaching skills extensively developed by Allen and Ryan (1969) can have a significant effect on changing the instructor's lecture-discussion performances. Allen and Ryan have divided the microteaching skills into the following five clusters representing 18 skills:

- Response repertoire
- Questioning skills
- Creating student involvement
- Increasing student participation
- Presentation skills

Of the 18 microteaching skills, only three skills will be discussed here: set, questioning skills, and reinforcement. These three skills were chosen because effective use of these skills will greatly improve the instructor's ability to successfully use the lecture-discussion.

**Set.** The term "set" refers to the response system that predisposes an individual to view or approach a situation in a predetermined manner. The actions that evoke a set are referred to as "set induction" in learning psychology. The concept of set induction is derived from the learning research that indicates activities preceding a learning task will influence the outcome of that task. Bruner (1966) argues that a set is one of the conditions that favor discovery learning.

The provision of a set at the beginning of a lecture-discussion motivates the student and establishes a link between the set induction and the instructional sequence to follow.

Techniques for providing a motivational set can vary — from the use of a "trigger" film to the use of a brief dramatic sentence. Examples of set induction follow.

**Examples**

An instructor, desiring to involve the class in a discussion of overpopulation, asks the class of 50 students to meet in a small seminar room furnished for 15 students. This experience is followed by a general discussion of the issues and problems relative to birth control in third world nations.

A short trigger film is shown of an elderly woman shoplifting while grocery shopping with a limited amount of money. After reviewing the film, the instructor and class explore the nutritional needs of the elderly, and the instructor concludes the lecture-discussion by asking the students to plan a low-cost, nutritional weekly menu for a healthy elderly woman on a limited budget.

Articles on child abuse, Medicare and Medicaid, poison control in pediatrics, or burn care — the list is only limited by the imagination of the instructor — are provided by the instructor before the class and instructor launch into a discussion of the topic chosen.

The instructor asks students to take notes with their left hands if they are right-handed and, conversely, to take notes with their right hands if they are left-handed. Then the instructor begins a lecture on the psychomotor rehabilitation required after a diagnosis of a cerebrovascular accident and resulting right hemiplegia.

To introduce a lesson on homeostasis, an instructor immerses a student's arm in a large bucket of ice cubes and directs the students to record the student's body temperature before and after immersion of the arm. This experience is followed by a lecture on the general principles of homeostasis.

A preinstructional set is exciting to use in the classroom. It can motivate students and provide a clue to the lecture-discussion to follow. Set induction serves as a reference point through which the instructor communicates to the student the context of the main body of the lesson. A set may be used at the beginning of the lecture-discussion or whenever the objectives of the lesson are changed. It also may be used to link units of instruction.

**Questioning skills.** Questioning, skillfully used, can assist students in exploring relationships, developing concepts and principles, analyzing and synthesizing information, and transferring knowledge. Questions permit students and teachers the opportunity through intensive interaction to explore the known and unknown together. The art of questioning is crucial to the skill repertoire of a good instructor.

There are several kinds of questions. Factual, descriptive, clarifying, higher-order, and divergent questions are discussed.

*Factual questions* require students to recall previously learned information. They are the easiest kind of question to ask and answer. The following are examples of factual questions.

**Examples**

What is the primary use of the drug metaraminol bitartrate (Aramine)?
What chamber of the heart receives venous blood from body tissues?
What food is a good source of potassium?

*Descriptive questions,* like factual questions, require students to recall information. However, they differ from factual questions in that they require students to organize their response in a logical manner and to respond with a more comprehensive answer. The following are examples of descriptive questions.

**Examples**

How would you describe the body posture children characteristically assume when they are seriously ill with meningitis?
How would you explain the differences between natural immunity, passive immunity, and active acquired immunity?
What public health measures help control the spread of tuberculosis?

*Clarifying questions* help the student to go beyond a superficial response to a more complete response. Questions may bring about clarification by asking for more information, requiring the student to defend the response, prompting or cuing the student, and/or redirecting the question.

**Examples**

What did you mean when you said that Mr. Jones was acting "strange"?
What are your reasons for strongly supporting sterilization for women after the age of 35?
If anti-inflammatory therapy is recommended for children with rheumatic fever, what would be the most likely prescribed drug?
Janet has stated that room temperature may be the cause of Mr. Madison's cold feet. Thomas, what might be another plausible reason?

*Higher-order questions* require students to go beyond factual knowledge — to do more than merely recall answers. They assist students to develop concepts and principles, transfer knowledge, draw inferences, and evaluate decisions. Higher-order questions seek evaluations, ask for inferences, and ask for comparisons.

• *Asking for evaluations.* Questions requiring evaluations imply that the students set up standards to use in answering the question.

**Example**

How would you evaluate a patient care plan based on described procedures for planning nursing interventions?

• *Asking for inferences.* Inferences involve either deduction or induction. Deduction is reasoning from a generalization or principle to a specific case. For example, the following is a deductive question.

**Example**

Mrs. Maria Campalli is a 59-year-old Italian patient with diabetes mellitus. What menu would you plan that still includes pasta products as part of her diet?

In contrast, inductive questions require the student to develop a generalization from a collection of specific facts or examples. For example, a student may be asked to record all the verbal and nonverbal responses of all newly admitted pediatric patients. From these observations, the students would be asked to make generalizations in regard to anxiety.

• *Asking for comparisons.* Comparison questions require students to determine if ideas, events, symptoms, and so forth are similar, dissimilar, unrelated, or contradictory. Examples of questions that seek comparisons follow.

**Examples**

What is the comparison between addiction to narcotics and alcoholism?
What are the contrasts between a cesarean section and a normal labor and delivery?
What is the relationship between diet and phenylketonuria (PKU)?

Higher-order questions may also require students to apply concepts and principles, problem solve, and determine cause and effect. Applying concepts and principles often requires deductive reasoning; determining cause-and-effect relationships often requires inductive reasoning.

Although higher-order questions require an in-depth knowledge of the subject matter and are difficult to construct and to answer, they can significantly enhance the quality of the lecture-discussion.

*Divergent questions* are probably not asked very often in the process of nursing instruction, because of the necessity of covering such a large amount of cognitive information. The divergent question has also been referred to as the "heuristic" or "creative" question. It has no "right" answer.

As an open-ended question, it allows the student freedom to explore problems, hypotheses, and the unknown. The following are examples of divergent questions.

### Examples

What might happen if all couples were limited by law to only two children?
What might happen if organ transplants were limited to individuals less than 21 years old?

**Reinforcement.** To successfully employ questioning skills, the instructor must be able to use reinforcement. The instructor's role as a positive reinforcer is crucial to increasing student participation in the classroom. If a student responds in a desirable manner, immediate positive reinforcement will increase the probability of the behavior being repeated. The difficulty with effectively using reinforcement is that no instructor can determine what will reinforce each individual student.

Four kinds of positive reinforcement can be used during lecture-discussion (Allen and Ryan, 1969):

1. *Positive verbal reinforcement.* This occurs when the instructor immediately follows a desired response with statements that indicate satisfaction with the response, such as: "I like your thinking on that issue!" "Good." "Excellent" "That shows exceptional insight."

2. *Positive nonverbal reinforcement.* This occurs when the instructor immediately follows a desired response with a nonverbal message that indicates satisfaction with the response: eye contact, affirmatively nodding the head as the student speaks, moving toward the student, and writing the response on the board are all examples of nonverbal reinforcement.

3. *Qualified positive reinforcement.* This occurs when the instructor reinforces only the correct part of the response.

### Example

INSTRUCTOR: Erica, what is the most characteristic sign of rubeola?
ERICA: I think it relates to a change of the mucosa of the mouth.
INSTRUCTOR: You're right, it is related to oral mucosa. What can be observed on the mucosa of the mouth?

4. *Delayed reinforcement.* This occurs when the instructor refers to a student's previous response.

### Example

INSTRUCTOR: Rheumatic fever is frequently classified as one of the collagen diseases. Sandra, in which body tissue is a pathologic condition observed when a collagen disease is present?
SANDRA: Muscular tissue. (The class is divided.)
INSTRUCTOR: Sandra, do you remember Karen's rationale and procedure for most effectively minimizing the joint pain resulting from rheumatic fever?

SANDRA: Yes. Karen recommended immobilizing the affected joints.
INSTRUCTOR: Excellent recall! Does that give you a clue?
SANDRA: If joint pain is involved, it must be connective tissue.
INSTRUCTOR: Good deductive thinking.

Notice that the instructor reinforced both Sandra and Karen. The instructor drew the attention of the class to Karen's earlier contribution and praised Sandra for deducing the answer to the original question.

Obviously, reinforcement must be appropriate to the response given. Saying "excellent" to an average response is ridiculous. However, skillfully used, reinforcement increases student participation in the classroom.

### Group discussion

Group discussion is a teaching method best used to develop both depth and breadth of knowledge. It is not generally recommended for presenting new material.

One type of group discussion used frequently in nursing is the conference. The clinical conference is a typical example. During the clinical conference, a plan of care is developed after an in-depth study of a patient's case.

Successful leading of a group discussion requires the instructor to develop communication skills. In addition to use of attending behavior, paraphrasing, reflection of feeling, and summarizing content, Taba (1967) suggests four additional communication skills for effective discussions:

1. *Focusing.* Through skilled use of a set, the instructor can help the group focus on the specific task.
2. *Refocusing.* This is often necessary when the group has strayed from the original topic.
3. *Changing the focus.* When the group has obviously exhausted the topic, changing the focus is necessary.
4. *Recapping.* Recapping, or summarizing, helps students draw relationships and understand the implications of the discussion.

Discussions are effective for changing attitudes, values, and behaviors. Their use often improves students' attitudes toward their instructor and their peers.

However, group discussions are often characterized by lack of direction. To help avoid this, some procedure must be developed to help adequately discuss the material. The Group Cognitive Map (Hill, 1977) is a procedural tool that outlines an orderly sequence that a group may follow to maximize the benefits of this teaching strategy. Use of the Group Cognitive Map assumes everyone has read all the required materials before the discussion; pooling ignorance is not group discussion.

The Group Cognitive map is made up of the following nine steps (Hill, 1977):

| Step | Name | Rationale and behavior |
|------|------|------------------------|
| 1 | Definition of terms and concepts | Mastering technical language is often an objective of nursing courses. For this step the instructor may wish to have medical dictionaries available. |
| 2 | General statement of author's message | This step provides a verbal abstract of the author's overall message (or messages). |
| 3 | Identification of major themes or subtopics | This step provides an analysis of the material into its constituent elements. Often the relative hierarchy of ideas is made clearer. The analysis clarifies communication and indicates how the communication is organized. |
| 4 | Allocation of time | This is a crucial step. Reasonable time limits set by group consensus help ensure both depth and breadth of coverage. The instructor must be prepared to monitor the allocation of time, no easy task. |
| 5 | Discussion of major themes | The emphasis is completely on a full discussion of the author's message (or messages) and not on personal opinions of group members. This is not to devalue personal opinions but rather to focus on what authorities in a field are saying. This important step is often completely eliminated in many group discussions. If this step is skipped, a discussion on unionization of nurses may degenerate into an exchange of personal opinions that leads to diversions and disagreement before the history, rationale, and pros and cons of the topic have been explored. |
| 6 | Integration of material with other knowledge | This step requires group members to make a conscious effort to transfer principles and concepts acquired in previous learning to a new situation. |

| Step | Name | Rationale and behavior |
|------|------|------------------------|
| 7 | Application of the material | Like step 6, this step requires members to make a conscious effort to assess the possible applications and implications of the material. |
| 8 | Evaluation of the author's presentation | This step finally allows for the personal opinions and reactions of the students. The previous steps have aided the student in the development of critical thinking and may have helped decrease affective loading. |
| 9 | Evaluation of group and individual performances | For discussion to continue successfully, this step is necessary. A knowledge of group processes, including group roles and member skills, is desirable to adequately evaluate group and individual performances. |

### Role playing

Role playing is an action technique in which two or more people first act out a realistic problem by drawing on information they are given, then follow up with a group discussion of the experience. The purposes are varied; however, for classroom teaching it is often used (1) to give insight into the attitudes and motives of others; (2) to create an awareness of how each student affects others; and (3) to develop skills in selected interpersonal processes.

For the first two purposes of role playing, the situational outcome is secondary to the student's ability to perceive the feelings, attitudes, and intentions inherent in the characters played.

For the third use of role playing—that of developing interpersonal skills (such as the affective skills of expressing empathy, expressing positive regard, reducing threat, and developing trust) and communication skills (such as attending behavior, paraphrasing, reflection of feeling, and summarizing content),—the situational context is of primary importance. The success of the role playing will depend on the student's ability to apply these interpersonal skills.

Immediately following the role playing, the process is analyzed and discussed. For instructors to optimally serve as discussion leaders, they need to have skills in observation, analysis, and group dynamics. The use of discussion is a critical component of this teaching technique.

Role playing promotes the intellectual, emotional, and physical involvement of the student, stimulates creativity, and maintains student interest. Role playing may be (1) open-ended (players are only given a problem and role), (2) structured (greater detail is provided in regard to the problems and roles), or (3) directed (a word-for-word script is provided). As already noted, role playing is very effective for affective learning.

### Demonstration

Demonstration is often the method chosen to teach psychomotor skills. Demonstration is a useful teaching method because it provides a complete sequence of behaviors necessary to perform a skill. De-Cecco (1968) discusses the following five basic steps necessary to teach a skill:
1. Analyze the skill by completing a task analysis.
2. Assess the entering behavior of students.
3. Arrange for training.
4. Describe and demonstrate the skill.
5. Provide opportunity for practice and feedback.
The last step is crucial to learning a psychomotor skill. A demonstration that does not include a practice component does not teach process; it merely presents cognitive content.

### Laboratory method

In the laboratory method, the student uses raw data for solving a problem. The process is usually divided into three stages: (1) an introductory stage, in which objectives are set and work is determined; (2) an actual laboratory or work period; and (3) a final stage, in which results are organized and findings are presented.

In its purest form, the laboratory method represents a research methodology. When applied to graduate nursing education, the laboratory method has two primary objectives (Stevens, 1976):
1. To teach research methodology.
2. To develop new nursing theory.
The clinical patient care assignment is an application of the laboratory method. In the introductory phase, the patient's current health status is assessed, and plans for nursing interventions are solidified. Then, the patient care plan is implemented. Finally, the nursing interventions are evaluated on the basis of predetermined objectives and standards.

A more obvious example of the laboratory method is the completion of an experiment in a science course such as genetics, biology, or chemistry. In the experiment, the objective, work activity, and results are held constant. Both cognitive and psychomotor learning are considered simultaneously.

### Independent study

Independent study provides an avenue for individualizing instruction. It seems to work best for students who are less rigid, have less need for social support, and have high achievement needs (Sorensen, 1968). It usually involves the completion of a project that a student has undertaken in order to gather and integrate data relative to some problem.

### Individualized instruction

Nursing schools are beginning to place greater emphasis on the development of individual responsibility for learning and intellectual inquiry. Individualized instruction permits a greater recognition of individual differences, for example, in students' learning rates. Some techniques currently being used to facilitate individualized instruction are auto-tutorial instruction, programmed instruction, and computer-assisted instruction.

**Auto-tutorial instruction.** The auto-tutorial method of instruction uses a multisensory approach with audio aids and media. The media may include tangible items, such as a hypodermic syringe; printed materials, such as textbooks, journal articles, and study guides; and visual aids, such as slides, films, and photographs.

The auto-tutorial method has some advantages over traditionally taught courses (Postlethwait and Mercer, 1972, Postlethwait, Novak, and Murray, 1972):

- The amount of repetition necessary for learning may be determined by the student.
- The amount of time necessary for learning may be determined by the student.
- The integration of cognitive information with learning activities is accomplished by the student with learning activities that require application of this knowledge.
- Students already possessing the required knowledge may pretest out of instruction.
- Instruction is standardized.
- Students become responsible for their own learning.

Although auto-tutorial instruction has several advantages, its primary limitation is the time required to plan and prepare the instructional sequence. Also, it is often very expensive.

A consistent finding in the research studies concerning auto-tutorial instruction is that the average time necessary to master similar course objectives by the auto-tutorial method is significantly less than the time needed with other instructional methods (Asklung, 1976, Pullon and Miller, 1972, Rutan, 1973, Thompson, 1972).

**Programmed instruction.** Programmed instruction is a method in which information is arranged in a series of sequenced steps, with testing and feedback at the end of each frame.

Two types of programmed instruction are most frequently used: (1) the linear model and (2) the branching model. The linear model provides only one set of exercises for all students to follow; consequently, all students respond to identical frames. In contrast, the branched model allows the student to proceed until a mistake is made or additional assistance is needed. When this happens, the student is instructed to branch to supplementary information that will aid in understanding the information being presented. The frames are generally longer in the branched program.

Programmed instruction is basically Skinner's (1954) research relative to operant conditioning applied to the classroom. Skinner argues that current educational practices are primarily dominated by aversive stimulation, that there is too great a time lapse between behavior and reinforcement, that skillfully developed programs of learning that move through a series of progressive approximations to final complex behaviors are lacking in many classrooms, and that reinforcement of desired behavior occurs too infrequently.

Skinner presented the following as primary advantages of programmed learning:

- Reinforcement of correct answers is immediate.
- Traces of earlier aversive control can be erased.
- An instructor can supervise an entire class; however, students may progress at their own rates.
- Students who are forced to leave school for personal reasons can return and continue where they left off.
- Through carefully designed instructional materials, instructors can arrange learning in a serial order and help students understand complex material.

**Computer-assisted instruction.** Computer-assisted instruction (CAI) is a result of the impact of the technological revolution on education. Basically, a CAI system includes a computing center and a number of student terminals. Typically, the student interacts with the stored instructional sequence by means of a typewriter keyboard or videoscreens that react to a light pen. The computer may communicate with the student by video or audio systems, or both.

The simplest model of a CAI system is similar to a linear programmed text, with the possible addition of an analysis of the students' answers at the end of the instructional sequence. It can be used to provide drill and practice. Donabedian (1976) describes the use of a CAI unit as a supplement to a traditionally taught lecture course in epidemiology. The computer-assisted instructional program supplements the lecture material by reinforcing and repeating the concepts presented in the lecture. The interaction is of a linear nature.

A second application of CAI is similar to a branching programmed text. Welch and associates (1977) describe the use of CAI to simulate a clinical encounter. Through the use of CAI, students are given a simulated patient history. Each student reviews the history and completes a pretest to determine his or her ability to recall significant information relative to the patient's history. After an intensive interaction between the CAI unit and the student, the student is required to give an analysis of the patient's problem, develop a treatment plan, and complete a posttest.

After the completion of the instruction and testing, the computer provides a printout of the complete interaction, including an analysis of the student's answers. The printout can then be used for student/teacher conferences.

Harless and associates (1971) describe a highly sophisticated application of CAI. This involves using a computer for the inquiry function. Basically, the computer acts as a human patient to simulate a clinical experience. The medical student is initially provided with a limited amount of patient information. The student must then order relevant diagnostic tests and ask questions to determine a diagnosis. The student's success is based on his or her ability to successfully diagnose. At the completion of the interaction, each student is provided with a printout that contains an analysis of the related questions asked, a list of the number of diagnostic tests ordered, and a summary of the unrelated interactions. This instruction is an integral part of the course.

Goroll (1977) describes another complex computer-assisted instructional program used to provide a wide variety of interaction. It also provides a significant portion of the course content.

Although CAI is still not readily used in nursing education, partly because of the lack of computer programs (software) and partly because of the expense of electronic equipment (hardware), it will most likely be increasingly developed for nursing instruction.

## Media

Media can be grouped into six classes: print, audio, still visuals, motion visuals, human interactions, and concrete objects. For the selection of media, the characteristics of the learner, the task, and the media must all be considered. Course objectives and content characteristics are also factors in media choice.

Historically, the nursing instructor and textbook have been the

**Table 1-1.** Media categorized by student response modality

| Listening/viewing | Reading | Interacting |
|---|---|---|
| Audiotape | Book | Skill practice |
| Slidetape | Periodical | Problem solving |
| Videotape | Programmed | Question exercises |
| film | instruction | |
| Demonstration | Chalkboard | Experiments |
| Concrete | Study guide | Computer-assisted |
| objects | Case study | instruction |

media of choice, with audio or visual aids used in limited fashion. However, the variety of media readily available to nursing instructors is considerable. Table 1-1 shows the most obvious media choices in the categories of listening/viewing, reading, and interacting.

In regard to the appropriateness of audiovisual aids, Davies (1973) has reviewed the research and concludes that learning from audiovisual aids can be effective. Furthermore, learning can be enhanced if instructors (1) state the objectives to be met by the media, (2) encourage student participation, and (3) use the media to repeat and reinforce previously learned information.

The medium selected should depend on the learning objectives to be met. Davies summarizes major trends from the research literature and concludes that:

- Cognitive objectives can be realized with all types of audiovisual aids.
- Affective objectives can be achieved most successfully through the use of still pictures, films, television, and audio aids.
- Psychomotor objectives can be achieved most successfully through the use of audio aids, large models of reality, and field trips.

In selecting a medium, the instructor should also keep in mind the principles of learning. Appropriate media will aid in the transfer of learning; provide reinforcement of the knowledge, skills, and attitudes to be learned; and assist in retention of knowledge.

After the selection of appropriate learning strategies, which incorporates the selection of methods and media, instruction can be implemented.

## POSTASSESSMENT

Postassessment is simply the means by which quantitative changes in behavior are observed with some degree of accuracy. The central questions are: What changes in behavior took place as a result of instruction? How can these changes be measured? The value of educational measurement depends on the validity of the answers to these questions.

Although this book is primarily concerned with the most technical aspects of test construction, it should be recognized that assessment provides direction for restating objectives, replanning preassessment instruments, and replanning learning strategies. In this broad interpretation, all the functions of postassessment are concerned with the facilitation of learning.

In the systems model, educational measurement is conceived not as a process apart from instruction but as an integral part of instruction. Without adequate postassessment, the instructor has no way of validating judgments regarding the effective selection of objectives and learning strategies.

Postassessment can facilitate learning when the following conditions are met:

- The outcomes selected for testing mirror the stated objectives of the nursing program. For example, if the instructional unit focuses on problem solving in nursing practice, the testing program must measure the student's ability to problem solve.
- Achievement testing is planned and developed as an integral part of the program of curriculum and instruction. When tests are selected and constructed in terms of the instructional program, with the results used to provide immediate feedback for instructional revision, their value cannot be questioned. In contrast, testing may be viewed with suspicion when it occurs merely as a parallel activity to instruction.
- Nursing instructors take an active role in the construction and development of all tests. Then, the testing program is under the direction and control of those responsible for instruction.

Postassessment can have a profound influence on the improvement of instruction; however, to do so, it must be seen as an integral part of the teaching/learning system, and the results must be used continuously to guide changes in the system.

Perhaps the most important outcome of evaluation is that it enables the instructor to identify with some confidence the strengths and weaknesses of the teaching and learning and to plan changes in the system to correct the weaknesses.

## INSTRUCTIONAL REVISION

The goal of nursing education is the attainment of specified outcomes—skills, knowledge, and attitudes. In order to accomplish these outcomes, strategies must be developed that identify weaknesses in teaching and learning. More important, we must be capable of and committed to beginning again. We must be open and flexible to change — not change for the sake of change but planned change based on reliable findings. As we return to that which was successful and discard that which was unsuccessful, we continually contribute to a nursing education program with sound objectives, effective teaching strategies, and competent entry-level professionals.

## REFERENCES

Allen, D., and Ryan, K.: Microteaching, Reading, Mass., 1969, Addison-Wesley Publishing Co.

Asklund, M., and others: Slide-tape versus lecture demonstration presentation of thermal agents in a physical therapist assistant program, Physical Therapy **56:**1361-1364, 1976.

Ausubel, D. P.: Educational psychology; a cognitive view, New York, 1968, Holt, Rinehart & Winston, Inc.

Bandura, A., and Walters, R.: Social learning and personality development, New York, 1963, Holt, Rinehart & Winston, Inc.

Bloom, B. S., editor: Taxonomy of educational objectives, handbook 1; the cognitive domain, New York, 1956, David McKay Co.

Bruner, J. S.: Toward a theory of instruction, Cambridge, Mass., 1966, Harvard University Press.

Canfield, A. A., and Lafferty, J. C.: Learning styles inventory manual, Plymouth, Mich., 1974, Elm.

Cohen, A. M.: Objectives for college courses, Beverly Hills, Calif., 1974, Glencoe Press.

Davies, I. K.: Competency based learning; technology, management and design, New York, 1973, McGraw-Hill Book Co., Inc.

DeCecco, J. P.: The psychology of learning and instruction; educational psychology, Englewood Cliffs, N. J., 1968, Prentice-Hall, Inc.

Donabedian, D.: Computer taught epidemiology, Nursing Outlook **24**(12):749–751, 1976.

Gagne, R. M.: The conditions of learning, ed. 2, New York, 1970, Holt, Rinehart & Winston, Inc.

Goroll, A. H.: Teaching differential diagnosis by computer; a pathophysiological approach, Journal of medical education **52:**153-154, 1977.

Harless, W. G., and others: Case; a computer-aided simulation of the clinical encounter, Journal of Medical Education **46:**443-448, May 1971.

Heidgerken, L. E.: Teaching and learning in schools of nursing; principles and methods, Philadelphia, 1965, J. B. Lippincott Co.

Hill, W. F.: Learning thru discussion, Beverly Hills, Calif., 1977, Sage Publications.

Holcomb, J. D., and Garner, A. E.: Improving teaching in medical schools; a practical handbook, Springfield, Ill., 1973, Charles C Thomas, Publisher.

Krathwohl, D. R., Bloom, B. S., and Masia, B. B.: Taxonomy of educational objectives, handbook II; the affective domain, New York, 1964, David McKay Co.

Mager, R. F.: Preparing instructional objectives, Palo Alto, Calif., 1962, Fearon Publishers.

Mizell, A. P., and Bell, J. E.: A review of the literature. In Postlethwait, S. N., and others, editors: Exploring teaching alternatives, Minneapolis, 1977, Burgess Publishing Co., pp. 97-120.

Popham, W. J., and Baker, E. L.: Systematic instruction, Englewood Cliffs, N. J., 1970, Prentice-Hall, Inc.

Postlethwait, S. N., and Mercer, F.: Study guide; mini courses—what are they? West Lafayette, Ind., 1972, Purdue Research Foundation.

Postlethwait, S. N., Novak, J., and Murray, J. T.: The audio-tutorial approach to learning, Minneapolis, 1972, Burgess Publishing Co.

Pullon, P. A., and Miller, A. S.: Evaluation of method of self teaching laboratory portion of pathology, Journal of Dental Education **36:**20-22, November 1972.

Roueche, J. E.: A place to begin; a systems approach to instruction. In Ford, C. W., and Morgan, M. K., editors: Teaching in the health professions, St. Louis, 1976, The C. V. Mosby Co. pp. 1-8.

Roueche, J. E., and Pitman, J.: A modest proposal; students can learn, San Francisco, 1972, Jossey-Bass.

Rutan, F.: Comparison of self instruction and lecture demonstration in learning a physical therapy skill, Physical Therapy **53:**521-526, May 1973.

Segall, A. J., and others: Systematic course design for the health fields, New York, 1975, John Wiley and Sons, Inc.

Simpson, E. J.: The classification of educational objectives in the psychomotor domain, The Psychomotor Domain, vol. 3, Washington, D. C., 1972, Gryphon House.

Skinner, B. F.: The science of learning and the art of teaching, Harvard Educational Review **24:**86-97, 1954.

Skinner, B. F.: Contingencies of reinforcement, New York, 1969, Appleton-Century-Crofts.

Sorensen, G.: An honors program in nursing, Nursing Outlook **16**(5):59-61, 1968.

Stevens, B. J.: The teaching-learning process, Nurse Educator **1**(1):9-20, May-June 1976.

Taba, H.: Handbook for elementary social studies, Palo Alto, Calif., 1967, Addison-Wesley Publishing Co.

Thompson, M.: Learning; a comparison of traditional and autotutorial methods, Nursing Research **21:**453-457, September-October 1972.

Trimble, W.: Rabid innovators; the behavioral objectivists, Community College Review **1**(2):37-41, July-August 1973.

Welch, A. C., and others: Computer-simulated clinical encounters (pt. 2), Journal of the American Dietetic Association **70:**385-386, April 1977.

Wong, M. R., and Raulerson, J. D.: A guide to instructional design, Englewood Cliffs, N. J., 1974, Educational Technology Publications.

# 2

# Constructing classroom achievement tests

Nursing educators are in the business of changing behavior. The assessment of change must be made and the circumstances under which this change occurs must be determined in order to provide a basis for reporting student progress, for motivating students, for diagnosing learning difficulties of individual students or of the entire class, and for providing students with the psychological security of knowing where they are in the course. In addition, assessment, when properly used, requires the teacher to carefully evaluate his or her instructional effectiveness. It seems reasonable to employ the most accurate and objective means available to make these assessments. This means testing, and testing requires that nursing educators know basic test theory and its use in everyday classroom evaluation (Chase, 1974).

This chapter presents the necessary steps for constructing classroom achievement tests. Fig. 2-1 presents a systematic procedure for test development.

## DEFINING OBJECTIVES

The learning outcomes measured by a test should accurately reflect the instructional objectives of the unit or course or both. Consequently, the students should be able to identify all the important areas to be reviewed before they take a test.

Of course, some instructional objectives cannot be measured by paper-and-pencil tests. Most of our instructor-made paper-and-pencil tests are developed to measure only the intellectual outcomes in the cognitive domain.

Bloom (1956) presents a framework around which instruction can be built to appropriately assess the outcomes of teaching. He presents

Adapted from King, E. C.: Constructing classroom achievement tests, Nurse Educator 3:30-36, September-October, 1978.

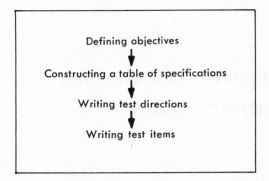

**Fig. 2-1.** Systematic procedure for test development.

six classes or categories of learning outcomes that are excellent guidelines for planning a course of study and evaluating that course of study. The six classes are outlined in Table 2-1. By starting with the relatively simple recall of information and proceeding to the increasingly complex levels of analysis, synthesis, and evaluation outlined in Table 2-1, we can write specific course objectives and plan for testing the specific outcomes of learning.

Some sample objectives for an obstetric nursing unit follow:
1. Describe the anatomical structure in which fertilization of the ovum normally occurs.
2. Describe the function of the placenta.
3. Plan a diet to avoid folic acid deficiency during pregnancy.
4. Formulate an exercise plan for a pregnant woman with diabetes who has lower back pain and varicose veins.
5. Discuss the rationale for showers rather than tub baths in late pregnancy.
6. Differentiate between true labor and false labor.
7. Explain the relationship between afterpains and breast-feeding the newborn.
8. Compare the immediate postpartum period of a heroin user with the same period in a nonheroin user.
9. Discuss the hazards that exist when the newborn has aspirated meconium.
10. Design a patient care plan for a newborn with hyaline membrane disease.

## CONSTRUCTING A TABLE OF SPECIFICATIONS

When learning outcomes have been well defined and the course content outlined, plans can be made for test construction. Good test

**Table 2-1.** Learning outcomes*

| Class or category | Measurable behavior | Verbs for use in writing objectives |
|---|---|---|
| 1.0 Knowledge (recalling previously learned material) | Defines terms; lists specific facts; states methodologies, principles, and rules. | Define, recall, name, list, repeat |
| 2.0 Comprehension (grasping the meaning of material) | Converts from one symbol system to another; explains material; and translates the material into own words. | Translate, discuss, describe, explain, recognize |
| 3.0 Application (using information) | Applies the appropriate abstraction without being prompted; interprets principles and rules as they apply to practice. | Interpret, illustrates, apply, use, demonstrate |
| 4.0 Analysis (breaking down material into its component parts) | Breaks down material into its component parts and compares the parts. | Analyze, differentiate, calculate, compare, contrast, categorize |
| 5.0 Synthesis (putting together parts to form a whole) | Produces something unique by restructuring and reordering ideas or objects. | Compose, rearrange, design, create, formulate |
| 6.0 Evaluation (judging the value of ideas works, solution, methods, materials, and so on) | Critically evaluates ideas, plans of actions, products, and so on, based on definite criteria. | Evaluate, assess judge, rate, appraise |

*Data from Bloom, B. S., editor: Taxonomy of educational objectives, handbook 1; the cognitive domain, New York, 1956, David McKay Co.

development begins with the development of a table of specifications (sometimes called "test blueprint"). This is a two-way table with subject matter content on one side and item type on the other. It has three purposes:
1. To establish the content for the test.
2. To balance test items among the instructional objectives.
3. To avoid loading the test with factual content and neglecting higher mental processes.
Since nursing instructors make decisions concerning student perfor-

**Table 2-2.** Table of specifications for a unit test on obstetric nursing

| Content | Knowledge | Comprehension | Application | Analysis | Synthesis | Evaluation | Summary |
|---|---|---|---|---|---|---|---|
| | | | | Outcomes | | | |
| Anatomy and physiology of the reproductive system | 10 (10%) | 5 (5%) | 5 (5%) | 0 | 0 | 0 | 20 (20%) |
| Pregnancy | 10 (10%) | 5 (5%) | 1 (1%) | 1 (1%) | 1 (1%) | 2 (2%) | 20 (20%) |
| Labor and delivery | 10 (10%) | 5 (5%) | 0 | 0 | 0 | 5 (5%) | 20 (20%) |
| Postpartum period | 10 (10%) | 2 (2%) | 3 (3%) | 1 (1%) | 1 (1%) | 3 (3%) | 20 (20%) |
| Care of the newborn | 10 (10%) | 5 (5%) | 0 | 1 (1%) | 2 (2%) | 2 (2%) | 20 (20%) |
| | 50 (50%) | 22 (22%) | 9 (9%) | 3 (3%) | 4 (4%) | 12 (12%) | 100 (100%) |

mance at many cognitive levels, they need data at all levels. Table 2-2 is a sample table of specifications for a unit test in obstetric nursing.

The raw numbers in each space of the table indicate the number of test items to be devoted to each major area. For example, 20 test items will be written to evaluate the section on labor and delivery; however, of these 20 test items, ten will measure knowledge, five will measure comprehension, and five will measure the student's ability to evaluate.

The percentage of the content areas to be tested and the percentage of emphasis placed on knowledge, comprehension, application, analysis, synthesis, and evaluation are both illustrated in each cell of Table 2-2. Note that the total of the percentages for six classes of learning outcomes is 100% and the total of the percentages for the content areas is 100%. In Table 2-2 the instructor has decided to divide obstetric nursing into five sections: anatomy and physiology of the reproductive system, pregnancy, labor and delivery, postpartum period, and the care of the newborn. Each receives a weight of 20%, since two weeks of instruction will be spent on each topic. Of course, one might take issue with the nursing instructor's choice of sections to emphasize. For example, some instructors may believe the greatest emphasis should be placed on labor and delivery, whereas others may believe the postpartum period needs more emphasis. Given the instructor's weighting decisions, however, we cannot say that the test plan in Table 2-2 is inappropriate.

In summary, the development of a table of specifications allows the instructor to build classroom tests that go beyond the knowledge level and ensures that the test is representative of the objectives stressed in class. It provides a realistic view of the testing situation. In addition, it allows the nursing instructor to know what is actually being assessed and, perhaps more important, what is *not* being assessed. After using this procedure, more than one instructor has changed the scope of his or her interpretation of classroom tests. With constant revisions, one table of specifications may assist the instructor with the construction of tests for a number of years.

The following examples illustrate how test items for Table 2-2 can be constructed to measure cognitive learning outcomes:

**1.0 Knowledge**

All of the following are phases of the menstrual cycle *except:*
1. Follicular phase
2. Ovulation
3. *Conception*
4. Luteinizing phase

**2.0 Comprehension**

During labor with a vertex presentation, the appearance of meconium-stained amniotic fluid usually indicates:
1. Abruptio placentae
2. *Some fetal distress*
3. Premature rupture of the membranes
4. Placenta previa

**3.0 Application**

When the known blood group of the mother is O and the blood group of the child is A, the possible blood group or groups of the father is(are):
1. A only
2. *A and AB*
3. A and O
4. A and B

**4.0 Analysis**

What effect will an unusual amount of exercise have on a pregnant diabetic woman's daily insulin requirement?
1. *Increase need for insulin*
2. Decrease need for insulin
3. May increase or decrease need for insulin, depending on specific trimester
4. No effect

**5.0 Synthesis**

A pregnant woman who has diabetes begins to sweat excessively, has dilated pupils and impaired vision, and becomes extremely irritable. What would be the best action or actions to take?
   a. Give any food containing sugar
   b. Give fluids without sugar
   c. Maintain body temperature
   d. Withhold insulin
   e. Give fruit juice
1. b and c
2. *a, d, and e*
3. b and d
4. None of the above

**6.0 Evaluation**

Kimberly, an unmarried, 19-year-old college student, has recovered from a therapeutic abortion. She wishes to return to college. Her mother wants her to come home for the remainder of the semester. She is an only child. Kimberly talks to her

nurse about the problem. Which response best illustrates the nurse's responsibility?
1. Encourage Kimberly to take advantage of her mother's offer since it will be better for her physical welfare.
2. Assist Kimberly in exploring her true feeling about her abortion.
3. *Help Kimberly explore the advantages and disadvantages of both situations so she can make her own decision.*
4. Listen to Kimberly, but refuse to discuss the problem, since she must solve the problem alone.

## WRITING TEST DIRECTIONS

The directions for a test should be as simple and as complete as possible. For a teacher-made test, adequate and complete directions should include the following (Thorndike and Hagen, 1969):

• The number of questions on the test.
• The number of pages making up the test.
• The exact amount of time in the testing period.
• A statement indicating how to record the answers.
• A statement telling the student to inspect the test before beginning.
• A statement indicating whether to guess when in doubt.

Whereas it is the student's responsibility to take the test, it is the nursing instructor's responsibility to prepare adequate directions. For example, suppose that during collation a page of the test were omitted. Without complete directions, how is the student to know that there are really 50 test items, not 35? Or suppose the instructor had planned to allow two hours to complete the test, although the usual classroom time is one hour. Or suppose the student marked all the answers on the original test booklet when an answer sheet is required for computer scoring. Good directions are important, and they contribute to the overall reliability of the entire test. An example of properly written test directions follows:

### Test directions

For each question below, choose the best answer. Indicate your choice by filling in the space under the appropriate number or letter on the answer sheet. Be sure that the number of the question you are answering is the same as the question number on the answer sheet where you are indicating your choice. Answer every question, even if you are not completely certain that the answer you are giving is the correct one. Each correct answer is worth one point. There are 40 questions on this test. Examine your test booklet to see that it has the required number of questions.

Write your name on the line provided on the test booklet, and record your booklet number on the answer sheet in the space labeled "Grade." You have two hours to complete this test. Do you have any questions about what you are to do? Turn the page and begin. *Good luck!*

## WRITING TEST ITEMS

In constructing an achievement test to fit the table of specifications, the instructor has a variety of item types as possible choices. Here we consider only objective test items. An objective test item is one that can be scored in such a way that there is an obviously right or most correct answer.

Objective test items can be divided into two kinds: (1) "supply type" objective items require the student to provide words, numbers, or symbols (short-answer and completion test items), and (2) "selection type" objective items require the student to choose the correct response (true/false, matching, and multiple-choice test items).

### Supply-type test items

The supply-type test item has two major advantages: it minimizes the likelihood of correct guessing, and it is relatively easy to construct. However, it has major weaknesses. First, supply items usually only demand recall of basic factual information rather than complex learning. In addition, they are often difficult to score because of the variety of partially correct responses.

#### *Guidelines for writing supply-type test items*

1. *Design items to have only one correct answer, which is short and definite.*

   POOR: The nerve that may be blocked by drugs is the _____.
   BETTER: The nerve that may be blocked by drugs in order to facilitate child-
   birth is the _____.

   The poor item has several correct answers and thus is difficult to score. The better item is much more definite, and, consequently, it is less ambiguous for the student and less difficult to score.

2. *Avoid removing statements verbatim from textbooks or other sources.* Wholesale lifting of passages encourages the student to memorize selected content from the course readings and does not encourage the student to apply data and make generalizations. In addition, statements may be taken out of context, and the "correct" answer may be very difficult for the student to determine.

   POOR: Before administering the drug digoxin, the nurse must take the
   _____.

BETTER: Which pulse must be taken before administering the drug digoxin?

_____

In the poor example, a sentence taken directly from a textbook, it is difficult to decide on the correct answer. For example, the student may write any response from "the temperature" to "the blood pressure." The rewritten test item is much clearer, and, consequently, it is easier to interpret and score.

3. *Avoid eliminating so many words that a clairvoyant is needed to answer the statement.*

POOR: A male child was born with erythroblastosis fetalis. The mother was _____ and the father was _____.

BETTER: A male child was born with erythroblastosis fetalis. The mother's blood was Rh _____ and the father's blood was Rh _____.

Eliminating too many terms from a statement makes it difficult for the student to respond. The poor item completely loses meaning and may frustrate the student.

4. *Always indicate the units in which the answer is to be expressed.*

POOR: The duration action of regular insulin is _____.

BETTER: The duration action of regular insulin is _____ hours.

Indicating the units in which the answer is to be expressed clarifies the item for the student and makes scoring easier.

5. *Place blanks near the end of the statement, not near the beginning.*

POOR: _____ normally fills the subarachnoid space.

BETTER: The subarachnoid space normally is filled with _____.

The reason for placing the blank near the end of the statement is that it allows the student to read the complete question before responding.

## True/false test items

The true/false item has been widely used in teacher-made classroom tests. These items can be written fairly rapidly, a large amount of subject matter can be tested in a relatively short period of time, and scoring is fast and easy. However, the true/false test item has also been subject to much-deserved criticism. The items often test relatively unimportant pieces of information, they encourage guessing, and they are often ambiguous.

## Guidelines for writing true/false test items

1. *Write statements that are true or false without qualifications.*

   POOR: **T** F Insulin is an effective drug for the treatment of diabetes mellitus.
   BETTER: **T** F Insulin is used as an effective drug for the treatment of diabetes mellitus when oral hypoglycemics or diet control alone is unsuccessful.

   Each item should be true or false without qualifications. Many statements that are supposed to be true cause difficulty because the critically thinking student can think of exceptions or reasons why the statement is not universally true. Although the poor statement is keyed "true," the students with the most information know there are many cases where oral hypoglycemics and diet control alone are effective treatments for diabetes mellitus. Such students may mark the poor statement false.

2. *Avoid use of specific determiners such as* only, all, never *(usually found in false statements) or* generally, often, sometimes *(usually found in true statements).*

   POOR: **T** F In 1900, most deaths were caused by infections.
   BETTER: **T** F The three leading causes of death in 1900 were pneumonia, tuberculosis, and diarrhea.

   Students will probably mark the first item as true; however, the rewritten item clearly demands more knowledge for the student to answer correctly.

3. *Keep true/false items relatively short and restricted to one central idea.* Short statements increase the likelihood that the item is clear and reduce the possibility of a guessing game.

4. *If true/false items are used often, be certain that the percentage of true/false items is not constant from test to test.*

### Special true/false items

The true/false item tends to be free of most criticism and be most useful when it is based on some given material (for example, a chart or patient case study). An advantage of this kind of question is that it allows the instructor to more effectively evaluate the student's ability to analyze, synthesize, and evaluate.

**Example**

A 16-year-old boy ate the following food during a 24-hour period:

| Breakfast | Lunch | Dinner |
|---|---|---|
| 1 piece of cherry pie | 1 cup of black coffee | 1 glass of milk |
| | 3 hamburgers with | ½ cup of rice |
| | 3 buns (12 oz) | 9 oz of chicken |

**Lunch**

20 pieces of French
fried potatoes

In which of the following was his diet lacking?

| | | | | | | |
|---|---|---|---|---|---|---|
| T | F | 1. Calories | T | F | 5. Protein |
| T | F | 2. Iron | T | F | 6. Vitamin A |
| T | F | 3. Carbohydrates | T | F | 7. Vitamin C |
| T | F | 4. Niacin | T | F | 8. Calcium |

## Multiple-choice test items

The multiple-choice test item is one in which an incomplete statement is presented and a number of possible responses or options are given. The question or incomplete statement introducing the item is called the "stem." An incorrect answer is called a "distracter" or a "foil." Fig. 2-2 illustrates the parts of a multiple-choice test item.

The outstanding feature of the multiple-choice item is its versatility. All levels of the cognitive domain can be tested by this item. It can be quickly and easily scored. Its primary limitation is that the multiple-choice item is often time-consuming and difficult to build. However, its advantages far outweigh these limitations.

Since writing good multiple-choice items takes much time and thought, many nursing instructors do not allow their examinations to be freely distributed. Students are allowed to review the examinations

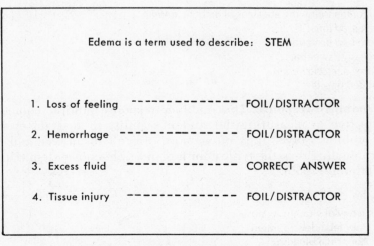

**Fig. 2-2.** Parts of a multiple-choice test item.

in the instructor's office. Consequently, the instructor does not have to completely rewrite examinations each semester.

### Varieties of multiple-choice items

**Negative.** There are many times when the use of negative wording is basic to the measurement of learning. For example, knowing that you should not administer a specific drug intravenously is so important it requires negative emphasis. Many nursing procedures place some emphasis on practices to be avoided. However, since negative expressions in the stem can present difficult reading problems to students, negative wording should be emphasized by underlining or the use of capital letters. Remember, the primary objective of testing is to measure learning outcomes, not to trick students.

**Example**

When one gives a hypodermic injection, all of the following are correct procedures
    except:
1. Withdrawing the needle quickly after the injection.
2. Cleansing the skin with an antiseptic before inserting the needle.
3. *Inserting the hypodermic needle at a ten-degree angle.*
4. Expelling air from the syringe before inserting the needle.

**Multiple-response.** In a multiple-response question, as few as one or as many as five correct answers may occur. To avoid possible confusion, you must write clear, concise directions if you use multiple-response items.

**Example**

Which of the following are signs of diabetic coma?
1. *Increased thirst*
2. *Increased urination*
3. Excessive sweating
4. *Fruity, acetone breath*
5. Dilated pupils

**Combined-response.** The combined-response multiple-choice item is effective in measuring the student's ability to analyze, evaluate, and problem solve. It is often more difficult to answer and more discriminating than the typical form of multiple-choice item (Hughes and Trimble, 1965).

**Examples**

A deficiency of vitamin A causes:
    a. Poor fetal development
    b. Abnormal bleeding

   c. Poor bone development
   d. Night blindness
   e. Skin disease
1. b and c
2. d only
3. *a, d, and e*
4. All of the above
Conditions in which cathartics are contraindicated include:
   a. Chronic constipation
   b. Bacterial infection
   c. Leukemia
   d. Post-myocardial infarction
1. a
2. a, b, and d
3. *c and d*
4. a, c, and d

### Guidelines for writing multiple-choice items

1. *Select foils that are plausible to those who do not know the content demanded by the item.*

   POOR: The caloric requirement of an 18-month-old infant is:
   1. The same as that of an adult male.
   2. Forty times that of an adult male.
   3. *About one-half that of an adult male.*
   4. Six hundred times that of an adult male.

   BETTER: The caloric requirement of an 18-month-old infant is:
   1. About the same as that of an adult male.
   2. *About one-half that of an adult male.*
   3. About two-thirds that of an adult male.
   4. About three-fourths that of an adult male.

   The revised item is obviously more difficult to answer than the original one, because the options are more plausible to those who do not know the content demanded by the item. In the poor example, the item really functions as a two-choice item, because no one is likely to choose options 2 or 4.

2. *Vary the number of available choices, using at least three, but not more than five.* We do not need to bluntly adhere to a fixed number of options for each multiple-choice item. Sometimes it is difficult to write four good foils. Rather than including a foil that is obviously incorrect, it is recommended to only use the most effective foils.

3. *Be certain that the length of the option is not related to the tendency to be correct.* There is a tendency for the correct answer

to be longer than the distracters because of the need to make the answer unequivocally correct. Obviously, this provides a clue to the test-wise student. If it is impossible to shorten the correct answer, adjust the distracters to make them approximately equal to length.

POOR: What determines the flavor, odor, appearance, and consistency of a fat?
1. Saturation
2. Nutrient content
3. *The particular fatty acid of which a fat is composed*
4. Hydrogenation

BETTER: What determines the flavor, odor, appearance, and consistency of a fat?
1. Saturation
2. Nutrient content
3. *Specific fatty acid*
4. Hydrogenation

4. *Place as much information as possible in the stem.*

POOR: In the article "The Medical Business" by J. L. Goddard, the author concludes that currently the Federal government has:
1. Adequate control over the manufacture of medical supplies.
2. *Little or no control over the manufacture of medical supplies.*
3. Very strict control over the manufacture of medical supplies.

BETTER: According to J. L. Goddard, what is the approximate amount of control the Federal government has over the manufacture of medical supplies?
1. Adequate control
2. *Little or no control*
3. Very strict control

By rewriting the poor item in question form, it is possible for the test-maker to avoid repeating material in each alternative. The improved item further clarifies the problem and reduces the time required to read the alternatives.

5. *Make all choices (correct answer and foils) grammatically consistent with the stem.* The correct response is almost always grammatically consistent with the stem. However, the instructor must take special care when writing the distracters. When the distracters are not grammatically consistent with the stem, test-wise students are likely to get the item correct without knowing the information.

POOR: In 1900, the leading causes of death were:
1. Accidents
2. Heart disease

    3. Cancer
    4. Typhoid fever and accidents
    5. *Infections and communicable disease*
BETTER: In 1900, the leading cause (or causes) of death was (were):
    1. Accidents
    2. Heart disease
    3. Cancer
    4. Typhoid fever
    5. *Infections and communicable disease*

6. *Make certain each item is independent of the other items.* Sometimes information is given in one item that helps to answer another item. These cues increase the likelihood that an alert student will obtain the correct answer without knowing the information. Sometimes instructors make the answer for one question depend on the correct answer to another question. Such interdependent items should also be avoided. They increase the likelihood that a student will answer correctly more items than his or her knowledge warrants.

## Matching items

The matching item is merely a modification of the multiple-choice item. Instead of testing the alternative responses beneath each individual stem, a series of stems, called *"premises,"* are listed in one column, and the responses are listed in a second column (Gronlund, 1968). The primary advantage of the matching item is that much factual information can be tested in a short time. However, good matching items are often difficult to build. Furthermore, all of the responses constructed for the test items must serve as plausible alternatives for each premise. If this does not occur, the matching item format is inappropriate.

### Guidelines for writing matching items

1. *Make lists of premises and responses as homogeneous as possible.* Unless all of the responses in the matching test item are reasonable alternatives to all of the premises, a matching item is not recommended.
2. *Write clear directions that specify if each response can be used once, more than once, or not at all.* Clearly written directions simplify the test item for the student and increase the overall reliability of the test.
3. *Arrange premises in logical order.* Dates should be arranged in chronological order; names of people, diseases, symptoms, and so on should be listed in alphabetical order.

4. *Keep responses short.* Short responses decrease the reading time and increase the probability that the responses are homogeneous.

POOR: Place the correct letter to the left of each answer:

| Column A | Column B |
|---|---|
| _____ 1. Aqueous humor | a. Between cornea and lens |
| _____ 2. Cochlea | b. Front of cerebrum |
| _____ 3. Iris | c. Forms part of boney labyrinth |
| _____ 4. Retina | d. Side of cerebrum |
| _____ 5. Temporal lobe | e. Circular colored disc |
| _____ 6. Frontal lobe | f. Back of cerebrum |
| _____ 7. Occipital lobe | g. Layer containing rods and cones |
| _____ 8. Parietal lobe | h. Middle of cerebrum |
| _____ 9. Pinna | i. External ear |
| _____10. Sclera | j. About 90% of outer eye |

BETTER: On the line to the left of each item in column A, write the letter (or letters) of the appropriate locations and functions listed in column B. Each item in column B may be used once, more than once, or not at all.

| Column A | Column B |
|---|---|
| a, e  1. Frontal lobe | a. Front of cerebrum |
| c, g  2. Occipital lobe | b. Side of cerebrum |
| d, f  3. Parietal lobe | c. Back of cerebrum |
| b, h  4. Temporal lobe | d. Middle of cerebrum |
| | e. Body movement |
| | f. Sensation |
| | g. Vision |
| | h. Hearing |

The poor example illustrates many of the common mistakes made in the writing of matching items: First, the directions are poor because they are not clear and do not specify the basis for matching. Second, the items in column A are heterogeneous. The better example has clear directions and a homogeneous column A.

## SUMMARY

This chapter is designed to help nursing instructors build better teacher-made tests. A systematic framework for test development that includes defining cognitive learning objectives; constructing a table of specifications; writing clear, concise test directions; and writing objective test items has been presented.

Improving their ability to write classroom achievement tests enables nursing instructors to more effectively monitor student progress,·

assess their own teaching effectiveness, and diagnose student learning difficulties.

By keeping in mind that test construction is a continuous process and by developing a systematic approach to test construction, we can produce superior classroom assessment instruments.

## REFERENCES

Bloom, B. S., editor: Taxonomy of educational objectives, handbook 1; the cognitive domain, New York, 1956, David McKay Co.

Chase, C. I.: Measurement for educational evaluation, Reading, Mass., 1974, Addison-Wesley Publishing Co.

Gronlund, N. E.: Constructing achievement tests, Englewood Cliffs, N.J., 1968, Prentice-Hall, Inc.

Hughes, H., and Trimble, W.: The use of complex alternatives in multiple-choice items, Educational and Psychological Measurement **25:**117-126, 1965.

Thorndike, R. L., and Hagen, E.: Measurement and evaluation in psychology and education, ed. 3, New York, 1969, John Wiley & Sons, Inc.

# 3

# The essay question

The most significant features of the essay examination are the freedom of expression and creativity allowed students and the emphasis on *depth* and *breadth* of knowledge.

The essay examination completely dominated classroom testing for the first third of the twentieth century. Advocates of the essay examination still believe it alone can measure the student's ability to employ higher mental processes to review his or her body of knowledge, to select the relevant concepts and principles, and to integrate them into a coherent whole. However, the mere administration of essay examinations does not ensure assessment of these abilities. Research has shown that essay tests, still widely used, should be used with considerable thought, planning, and preparation.

"The essay question is defined as a test item which requires a response composed by the examiner . . . of a nature that no single response or pattern of responses can be listed as correct, and the accuracy and quality of which can be judged subjectively only by one skilled or informed in the subject" (Stalnaker, 1963, p. 495). However, as empirical evidence clearly indicates, instructors, those skilled and informed in the subject, often disagree about the accuracy and quality of essay papers.

Classic studies by Starch and Elliott (1913) concluded that instructors cannot agree on what constitutes an acceptable essay answer, even in such an "objective" subject area as geometry. Diederich (1967), in a study conducted by the Educational Testing Service, also found that raters awarded each student's composition scores ranging from "failure" to "excellent." Levine (1976) found during a clinical psychology program evaluation that when experts were asked to score preliminary papers using a carefully developed rating scale, one student received an A from one expert and an unacceptable grade from a second.

In addition, Ashburn (1938) had college instructors read the same essays at two separate intervals. He found inconsistency between the two scores from the same instructor. Downie (1967) found that an in-

44

structor shows considerable variation in scoring a paper after a few months. Thus, reliability in scoring essay examinations is a serious limitation of this type of examination item.

Unreliability of scoring is influenced by a student's skill in written expression. Marshall and Power (1969) found that the student's handwriting influences the essay test grade. Studies by Gosling (1966) and Scannel and Marshall (1966) show that a grade is often affected by the student's skill in writing, spelling, and grammar. A student with little mastery of the subject matter but well-developed writing skill may thus receive a passing grade. Another student with little mastery of the subject matter and poorly developed writing skill may receive a failing grade. The difference between the students is not in subject matter mastery but in writing ability. Students with good writing skills get inflated grades. Scannel and Marshall found that writing ability influenced test scores even when graders were cautioned to disregard errors in punctuation, spelling, and grammar.

Variables related to the instructor also influence grading. Bracht and Hopkins (1968) found that grader fatigue influences essay scores. Papers that are read first receive higher scores than papers read toward the end of the grading session.

In general, research suggests that students who do well on essay tests also do well on objective tests. Of course, the relationship is not perfect, but it is fairly strong and positive. Godshalk, Swineford, and Coffman (1966), in a study supported by the College Entrance Examination Board, found a strong positive relationship between essay test scores and multiple-choice test scores.

In all fairness, it should be pointed out that some of the unreliability of scoring is a direct result of the absence of scoring guidelines or of a scoring key. Goldshalk, Swineford, and Coffman (1966) found that essay tests can be graded reliably when scoring rules are considered.

The use of restricted response essay questions also increases the reliability among graders (Grant and Caplan, 1957, Stalnaker, 1937). However, when a response is restricted, the student's freedom of expression is diminished. The item's power to demand that the student select, organize, and creatively communicate information is diminished. The instructor's ability to test the student's integration and organization of knowledge is also diminished. Thus, advantages of using essay test items are offset.

Differences can be illustrated between objective and essay test items. Five general characteristics useful in differentiating the items are presented in Table 3-1. The table shows that the use of both objective and essay test items balances a testing program.

**Table 3-1.** Comparison of objective and essay test items

| Trait | Objective test item | Essay test item |
|---|---|---|
| Abilities measured | Excellent for measuring knowledge, comprehension, application, and analysis. | Best for measuring analysis, synthesis, and evaluation. |
| Sampling | Representative sampling extensive. | Representative sampling limited. |
| Item preparation | Time-consuming and difficult. | Difficult, but easier than objective items. |
| Scoring | Simple, reliable, and fast; can be scored easily by computer. | Difficult, unreliable, and time-consuming; often requires a content expert for scoring. |
| Nature of student response | Student required to select response. | Student required to organize knowledge into a coherent whole. |
| Validity | Easy to obtain an uncontaminated measure of achievement. | Difficult to obtain an uncontaminated measure of achievement. |

## DESIGNING ESSAY TEST ITEMS

Essay tests have a legitimate place in the evaluation of student achievement. However, the instructor must make a conscious effort to understand the limitations of the item and to carefully design, write, and score the examination. These guidelines can hardly be overemphasized.

The learning outcomes measured by an essay test item should accurately reflect the instructional objectives of the learning unit or course. The essay test item is most useful for measuring higher-level cognitive learning. With reference to Bloom's (1956) taxonomy, this test item form is useful for assessing the student's performance in the areas of (1) analysis, (2) synthesis, and (3) evaluation. The table of specifications (see Chapter 2) will include essay items if they are needed to ensure thorough testing in these areas.

### Analysis

Analysis requires the ability to break down material into its component parts and to ascertain the relationships and organizing principles among those parts. Analysis includes (1) analysis of elements, (2) analysis of relationships, and (3) analysis of organization principles (Bloom, 1956).

Analysis of elements requires the student to infer unstated assumptions, identify important elements, distinguish between fact and opinion or hypothesis, and distinguish conclusions from the facts that support them. Analysis of relationships requires the student to recognize cause-and-effect relationships and distinguish between relevant and irrelevant arguments and facts. Analysis of organizational principles requires the student to infer the form or structure that is implicit in the communication. For example, the student might need to be able to infer a philosophy of education from reading the nursing school's mission statement.

Following are two examples of essay test items designed to assess the student's ability to recognize unstated assumptions (analysis of elements).

### Example

DIRECTIONS: Select the response (A, B, C, or D) that you believe is the most correct, and discuss the principle that supports your conclusion. If you believe the "best" response is inadequate, formulate a better one. Discuss the rationale for your improved response, and discuss the principle that supports your conclusion. For each of the three options you have *not* chosen, discuss the principle on which you rejected it.

> M. L., an elderly Navajo woman with a diagnosis of congestive heart failure, was convinced that only her medicine man could remove the evil causing her illness; otherwise she would die. Administrative arrangements were made for the ritual. Shortly after the ritual, the patient began to adhere to the medical regimen and improved physically and emotionally.

Which of the following statements assesses this situation most clearly?
A. Psychiatric consultation would have been more appropriate.
B. *Knowledge, decisions, judgment, and collaboration will equal desirable outcomes.*
C. Although superstitions should be assessed during the phases of the nursing process, they should not be reinforced in the medical regimen.
D. Adequate interactions between nurse and patient would have eliminated the need for a medicine man.

### Example

DIRECTIONS: Fill in the blanks below with the correct answers.

> A 26-year-old man has been supported with hemodialysis for 11 months. He admits chronic diet abuse and frequently gains large amounts of weight between dialyses. Such difficulties have evolved in part from marital diffi-

culties and have resulted in periodic episodes of severe congestive heart failure. He has been removed from the home dialysis program and admitted to a hospital. A 1.5 gram sodium diet restriction has been ordered.

1. Prepare a restricted sodium diet for two days.
2. Break down the diet, and include seasonings other than salt to add variety to the sodium-restricted diet.

| Date | Blood pressure (mmHg) | Weight on (kg) | Weight off (kg) | Total weight v (kg) | Daily weight (kg/day) |
|---|---|---|---|---|---|
| 11/3 | 148/80 | 58.7 | 55.7 | X | X |
| 11/6 | 144/86 | 59.6 | 55.7 | 1___ | 2___ |
| 11/8 | 160/100 | 58.2 | 3___ | 2.5 | 4___ |
| 11/10 | 154/80 | 5___ | 55.6 | 6___ | 0.5 |
| 11/13 | 166/84 | 7___ | 55.6 | 3.3 | 8___ |
| 11/15 | 144/90 | 57.9 | 55.5 | 9___ | 10___ |

## Synthesis

Synthesis requires the student to put together elements and parts in order to form a whole. This involves rearranging and combining parts to create a pattern or structure not clearly seen previously. Three components of synthesis have been proposed by Bloom (1956):

1. *Production of unique communication.* The development of communication in which the student attempts to convey ideas, feelings, and/or experiences to others: for example, a counseling response on a psychiatric nursing examination.
2. *Production of a plan or proposed set of operations.* The development of a plan of work or the proposal of a plan of operations, such as a patient care plan.
3. *Development of a set of relationships to explain data or phenomena.* The development of a hypothesis, such as an explanation to account for noncompliance with a nursing care plan on the part of an Italian-American or Chinese-American patient.

Since the process of synthesis places emphasis on creativity and organizational skills, essay test items play a major role in assessing objectives written for this level of learning.

Following are two examples of essay test items designed to assess the student's synthesizing skills.

### Example

Miss K. S. is an underweight, 19-year-old woman who enters the hospital with a three-month history of anorexia and nausea. Laboratory findings show the following:

| | |
|---|---|
| BUN | 150 mg/100 ml |
| Urinary sodium | 42 mEq/liter |
| Serum creatinine | 15 mg/100 ml |
| Blood pH | 7.45 |

1. What would you expect the diet order to be?
2. Justify any diet modifications indicated.
3. Determine the caloric intake of the modified diet.
4. Construct a sample menu plan for one day.

**Example**

Mrs. B. Y., an extremely apprehensive 45-year-old woman, mother of three teenaged children, has been admitted with irregular and heavy vaginal bleeding. Biopsies demonstrate the presence of squamous cell carcinoma and a poor prognosis. Following surgical insertion of radium, the patient becomes convinced that she has become radioactive and refuses any association with her concerned family. She has apparently decided that dying is preferable to living.

1. Discuss how each component of the nursing process relates to the care of this patient.
2. Discuss the specific skills necessary for successful completion of the nursing process as they relate to Mrs. B. Y. Directly relate the skills to the case study.

**Evaluation**

Evaluation requires students to make judgments concerning the value of material and methods. The most complex of cognitive behaviors, it requires students to make quantitative and qualitative judgments based on standards. Both the consciousness of the judgment and the use of criteria are essential (Bloom, 1956).

The essay test item is excellent for use as a comprehensive assessment of the student's skill in evaluating. Testing at this level requires that a complete work plan or proposal be given to the students. They would be required to (1) analyze it, (2) make judgments concerning it based on specified criteria, (3) synthesize the results into an overall evaluation, and (4) possibly make recommendations. Because of the time required for this process, the instructor may wish to assign such an item as a take-home examination.

The final evaluation may be made in terms of internal evidence or external criteria:

- *Internal evidence.* Evaluation may be based on internal standards such as accuracy of data, consistency, and logic.
- *External criteria.* Evaluation may be based on commonly accepted standards.

Students may be given the evidence or criteria, or they may be required to supply them.

Following are two examples of essay test items designed to assess the student's evaluation skills. The first requires the student to use internal evidence; the second, external criteria:

**Example**

DIRECTIONS: Given the following set of research papers in nursing and using the following internal evidence, judge each research paper and select three papers for presentation to the class.

Research paper: _____

| | Unacceptable | Below average | Average | Above average | Excellent | Does not apply |
|---|---|---|---|---|---|---|
| 1. Statement of problem | 1 | 2 | 3 | 4 | 5 | NA |
| 2. Statement of purpose | 1 | 2 | 3 | 4 | 5 | NA |
| 3. Outline of protocol | | | | | | |
| Description of subject (or subjects) | 1 | 2 | 3 | 4 | 5 | NA |
| Description of protocol | 1 | 2 | 3 | 4 | 5 | NA |
| 4. Description of findings | 1 | 2 | 3 | 4 | 5 | NA |
| 5. Conclusions and/or relationship of findings to purpose | 1 | 2 | 3 | 4 | 5 | NA |
| 6. Overall quality | 1 | 2 | 3 | 4 | 5 | NA |

TOTAL POINTS _____

A. State here your rationale for using any "does not apply" answer.

B. Comments:

**Example**

DIRECTIONS: Given the following set of research papers and using the following external criteria established for scoring preliminary papers, judge the acceptability of each research paper:

- Whereas all students are expected to strive to complete a paper that merits publication in a reputable professional source (for example, *Psychological Bulletin* or *Psychological Review*), it is not expected that all acceptable papers will achieve that standard. At the minimum, an acceptable paper will be one expected of a competent professional, able to amass, review, and evaluate evidence and draw appropriate conclusions about the state of knowledge or the state of the art in a given field.

- In judging the acceptability of a paper, the faculty member may consider as a standard whether or not the student could be recommended for a position requiring application of skills, at a beginning professional level, of the kind demonstrated in completing the paper. Although other factors (such as other experience with the student or nature of the position) would be weighed in the actual decision to write a recommendation, as set forth here the standard provides a mental guideline for the faculty member judging the acceptability of the paper.

## GUIDELINES FOR WRITING ESSAY TEST ITEMS

1. *Write test items in clear, precise language.*

POOR: Discuss the nursing care of Mrs. R. L. T., a 70-year-old woman with arteriosclerotic heart disease and congestive heart failure.

BETTER: Discuss the nursing care of Mrs. R. L. T., a 70-year-old woman with arteriosclerotic heart disease and congestive heart failure. Include the following in your discussion:
- Definition of arteriosclerosis and congestive heart failure.
- List of symptoms of arteriosclerosis and congestive heart failure.
- Description of expected abnormal laboratory results and x-ray film results.

Develop a nursing care plan to:
- Facilitate the provision of oxygen to all cells.
- Facilitate the maintenance of fluid and electrolyte balance.
- Decrease patient's anxiety and fear resulting from restricted activity.

Give the scientific basis for each nursing intervention.

The first item is much too broad and vague. The student is faced with many questions. Am I to consider initial treatment through discharge? What is Mrs. R. L. T. like? What are the medical orders? Am I only to describe the care or justify it as well? The second test item is much more definite. It also decreases the student's temptation to bluff.

2. *Write directions in clear, precise language.*

POOR: Answer the following question in as brief a manner as possible.

BETTER: Each of the following three questions is based on a case study from a psychiatric setting. Each case study includes three possible responses. Select the response you believe is best, and state the principle on which the response is based. The answer should be written in prose form. You will be graded on organization, depth of analysis, and presentation of relevant principles. You have three hours to complete the examination. Each question is worth 20 points.

A good set of directions should indicate:
- A general plan for attacking the test item.

- The form in which the answer should be written: prose or outline.
- Criteria that will be used for grading: If such factors as grammar, spelling, and handwriting are to be graded, the directions should say so. Use of such factors must be consistent with the course objectives, and these factors should be graded separately from content.
- The time available for taking the test.
- The point value of each test item: if the test includes a combination of essay and objective test items, mention the percent of the total grade that the essay items represent (Green, 1975, Thorndike and Hagen, 1969).

3. *Restrict use of essay items to assessment of higher-level cognitive skills.*

> POOR: List three drugs that help regulate electrolyte balance.
> BETTER: State the general category of each of the following drugs, and indicate one use for each drug. Discuss any dietary implications.

Objective test items are superior to essay test items for assessing knowledge, comprehension, and application of information. Problems of scoring and sampling should limit the use of essay items to measuring higher-level learning outcomes.

4. *Require all students to answer the same test item.* When students are allowed a choice of test items, the common basis on which different individuals may be compared when one uses the rating method of grading is lost. This further decreases the reliability of an item type that already has reduced reliability. Furthermore, because of the time required to adequately answer the essay test item, sampling of course material is severely limited. This sampling error reduces the content validity of a test whose content validity is already suspect.

In some testing situations, the use of optional test items may be defensible. If the class has pursued individual projects through independent study, optional items may be the only sensible solution.

5. *Provide adequate time for students to respond to each item.* The instructor should carefully consider the number and type of essay test items when determining the time for a test. Students need time to organize, outline, and integrate principles and concepts. If this time for thinking as well as writing is not provided, the essay test will not truly measure what it purports to measure. A high score may represent writing

speed rather than overall achievement of course objectives. The more complex the test item, the longer the time required.

## TYPES OF ESSAY TEST ITEMS

Whereas freedom of expression is one of the major advantages of the essay test item, the actual freedom permitted varies. Students may be required to construct precisely defined responses—"restricted" responses—, or they may be allowed great freedom in determining the nature and scope of their responses—"extended" responses (Ahmann and Glock, 1975).

### Restricted response essay items

The restricted response test item clearly defines the parameters of the student's response. It is often compared with the supply type of test item discussed in Chapter 2. However, the restricted response item is not confined to a few words, and it measures more complex achievement than the supply item. It is more easily scored than the extended response item but may provide less opportunity for students to demonstrate their ability to develop new patterns of response. It may also decrease the students' opportunities to demonstrate synthesis and evaluation skills.

#### Example

As a coronary care nurse, you observe the following on the electrocardiogram (EKG) monitor:
- Atrial premature contractions
- Atrial tachycardia
- Atrial flutter
- Atrial fibrillation

1. What medication would the doctor probably order?
2. Draw the structure of the medication, and explain its pharmacological effect on the myocardium.
3. Draw the four arrhythmias you saw on the EKG monitor and discuss their clinical significance.

### Extended response essay items

The extended response test item emphasizes the holistic approach. It is used to reveal information regarding the structure, dynamics, and functioning of a student's higher-level mental processes as they have been modified by a specified set of learning experiences (Sims, 1938). The most recurrent criticism of the extended response item is its scoring unreliability. Its practical value may be limited by the instructor's inability to score the item reliably. However, a *mixture of* extended and restricted response test items improves test reliability and enhances content validity. When extended and restricted response items are mixed, the higher reliability of the restricted response items will strengthen the overall test reliability.

The extended response item provides the student with almost unlimited freedom to determine the response, as the following examples reveal.

**Examples**

In what ways is psychotherapy inadequate?

How have psychotropic and other drugs affected the care of psychiatric patients? Has their use been beneficial or detrimental to psychiatric patients? Support your answer with documentation.

What are some of the major problems in adequately measuring the quality of health care?

## GUIDELINES FOR GRADING ESSAY TEST ITEMS

There are two basic procedures for grading essay items: (1) the analytical scoring method and (2) the rating method. With both methods it is recommended that papers be scored anonymously to avoid the "halo effect." This term refers to the tendency of instructors to base their evaluation of a test item on their general favorableness toward the person taking the test.

### Procedure for analytical scoring (Green, 1975)

1. Construct a scoring key. The scoring key should include the total point value for each test item and the relative point value for each part of the test item. This is illustrated in the following sample test item and answer key.

   TEST ITEM: Mr. Smith was admitted to the hospital with a complaint of severe shortness of breath. His vital signs on admission were: temperature, 101 F, pulse, 120, and respiration, 20. Mr. Smith has had chronic obstructive pulmonary disease for ten years. His arterial blood gas analyses shortly after admission showed:

   | | |
   |---|---|
   | pH | 7.24 |
   | $P_{CO_2}$ | 100 mmHg |
   | $P_{O_2}$ | 33 mmHg |

   The physician ordered oxygen to be delivered at 10 liters per minute continuously by face mask.

   What do you expect to happen to Mr. Smith shortly after he receives the oxygen? Using your knowledge of chemoreceptors, explain why this will happen. (15 points)

ANSWER KEY: Mr. Smith will probably become apneic. (5 points) The central chemoreceptors respond to the level of $CO_2$ in the arterial blood. However, if the $CO_2$ rises to extremely high levels, as in Mr. Smith's case (100 mmHg), the central chemoreceptors become insensitive and no longer stimulate ventilation. (3 points) The peripheral chemoreceptors primarily respond to $O_2$ levels in the arterial blood. With his central chemoreceptors insensitive, Mr. Smith's sole stimulus to breathe would be his peripheral chemoreceptors. Giving Mr. Smith oxygen will cause his $Po_2$ to rise, but his ventilation will not improve and permit his $Pco_2$ to decrease. (3 points)

Since his $Po_2$ is adequate after he receives the oxygen by mask, Mr. Smith's peripheral chemoreceptors would try to stimulate breathing. But since his $Pco_2$ is still extremely high, his central chemoreceptors will not stimulate ventilation. Therefore, Mr. Smith will not breathe. (4 points)

2. Score all answers to one test item at the same time. Scoring essay items one at a time increases the reliability of the scoring. It also helps reduce the halo effect in grading. When each answer is scored simultaneously, the instructor gets an overall impression of the range of abilities students show in responding to the test item. Repeat this procedure until the entire examination is graded.
3. Total the points on each paper and assign a final grade.

The analytical scoring method is recommended for restricted response essay items. It greatly increases scoring reliability.

## Procedure for rating

1. Construct a sample response. Extended response items permit much freedom in answering, and the preparation of a model answer is difficult but not impossible. After a model has been prepared, it should be checked against a sample of student responses. If it is found that the students consistently respond differently from the model answer, then the model answer should be revised. Some instructors object to this procedure on the grounds that it lowers academic standards. However, the discrepancy between responses may result from poor directions, a poorly designed test item (or items), or expectations that are unrealistic in light of students' previous learning or the limits of test time (Thorndike and Hagen, 1969).
2. Clearly state the criteria for evaluating the answer.
3. Read responses one at a time, sorting them into predetermined piles that represent the letter grades to be assigned. During this first reading, those answers that do not clearly fall into any

grade category should be identified with a question mark and placed in the most appropriate pile.
4. Reread each response, giving selected attention to the papers carrying a question mark.
5. Repeat steps 3 and 4 for each essay item.
6. If the item deals with a controversial issue, be especially careful to evaluate it in terms of the *presentation of evidence* for the position chosen, rather than the choice itself.
7. Shuffle the papers after scoring each response. The grading of a paper may be influenced by the quality of the previous response. For example, suppose Jennifer wrote a superior answer to each essay question. However, Jim's answers are average. If the instructor reads Jim's adequate but average responses after reading Jennifer's superior answers, Jim's answers may all appear below average. To prevent Jim's overall grade from being systematically lowered, the papers should be shuffled to vary the scoring sequence.
8. Tally the letter grades for each essay item and assign an overall letter grade.

The rating method is recommended for grading extended response essay items. However, it is not very reliable.

Whether using the analytical scoring method or the rating method, instructors should concentrate on correcting errors and writing comments on essay items. Carefully scored essay items maximize student motivation and learning. It is far better to carefully prepare and score one item than to cursorily score five. Carefully considered written comments can be another excellent mechanism for increasing student motivation. Thorough feedback is more effective than most instructors realize. It is like a private conversation between instructor and student and is highly valued by students.

## SUMMARY

The most significant features of the essay examination are (1) the freedom of expression and creativity allowed students, (2) the emphasis on depth and breadth of knowledge, and (3) its usefulness for measuring higher-level cognitive learning.

Since essay test items have a legitimate place in evaluating achievement, the nursing instructor must make a conscious effort to consider the recommendations for writing and scoring test items. When these recommendations or guidelines are considered, the overall test validity and reliability will be substantially improved.

## REFERENCES

Ahmann, J. S., and Glock, M. D.: Evaluating pupil growth, ed. 5, Boston, 1975, Allyn and Bacon.

Ashburn, R. R.: An experiment in the essay-type question, Journal of Experimental Education **7**:1-3, 1938.

Bloom, B. S., editor: Taxonomy of educational objectives, handbook 1; the cognitive domain, New York, 1956, David McKay Co.

Bracht, G. H., and Hopkins, K. D.: Objective and essay tests; do they measure different abilities? (paper presented at the annual meeting of the American Education Research Association, Chicago, 1968).

Diederich, P.: Cooperative preparation and rating of essay tests, English Journal **56**:573-584, 1967.

Downie, N. M.: Fundamentals of measurement, New York, 1967, Oxford University Press.

Godshalk, F. I., Swineford, F., and Coffman, W. E.: The measurement of writing ability, New York, 1966, College Examination Board.

Gosling, G. W. H.: Marking English compositions, Victoria, Australia, 1966, Australian Council for Educational Research.

Grant, L. D., and Caplan, N.: Studies in the reliability of short-answer essay examinations, Journal of Educational Research **51**:109-116, 1957.

Green J. A.: Teacher-made tests, ed. 2, New York, 1975, Harper and Row Publishers, Inc.

Levine, M.: A statement of purposes and standards for the preliminary paper requirement in the clinical-community area (minutes of jury trial to evaluate the clinical psychology program, State University of New York at Buffalo, June 1976).

Marshall, J. C., and Power, J. M.: Writing neatness, composition errors and essay grades, Journal of Educational Measurement **6**:97-101, 1969.

Scannel, D. P., and Marshall, J. C.: The effect of selected composition errors on grades assigned to essay examinations, American Educational Research Journal **3**:125-130, March 1966.

Sims, M.: Reducing the variability of essay examination marks through elementary variation in standards of grading, Journal of Educational Research **26**:637-647, 1938.

Stalnaker, J. M.: Essay examinations reliably ready, School and Society **46**:671-672, 1937.

Stalnaker, J. M.: The essay type of examination. In Lindquist, E. F., editor: Educational Measurement, ed. 5, Washington, D. C., 1963, American Council on Education, p. 495.

Starch, D., and Elliott, E. C.: Reliability of grading work in mathematics, School Review **21**:254-259, 1913.

Thorndike, R. L., and Hagen, E.: Measurement and evaluation in psychology and education, ed. 3, New York, 1969, John Wiley & Sons, Inc.

# 4

# Basic test attributes

Nursing educators are directly and substantially involved in both the development of assessment instruments and the use of standardized assessment instruments. Consequently, they are asked: Are the assessment instruments you are using valid? Are they reliable? Are they both practical and interpretable? These are the characteristics we all strive for. We want our tests to be accurate representations of the variables we are interested in measuring (for example, clinical performance or achievement in pharmacology). We want the test results to measure consistently, that is, remain stable over time. Finally, we want the tests to be easy to administer, economical, and easily interpretable.

## VALIDITY

"Validity" refers to the capacity of a test to measure what it purports to measure. For example, the Nursing Board Examination (NBE) score is valid to the extent it tells us the truth concerning an individual's ability to perform adequately as a nurse. A teacher-made test on diabetes mellitus is valid to the extent it tells us the truth concerning a student's knowledge relevant to the disease. *Validity* is technically defined as the correlation between test measures and criterion measures.

There are three basic types of test validity. Each type provides a different kind of information:

1. *Content validity* expresses the degree of relationship between the content of the test and the content of the course.
2. *Criterion-related validity* is concerned with the degree of relationship between test performance and other kinds of student performance observed either now (concurrent validity) or in the future (predictive validity).
3. *Construct validity* expresses the degree of relationship between test performance and the possession of psychological traits or qualities.

## Content validity

Content validity is the most important type of validity to consider when one analyzes teacher-made tests. An assessment of content validity is primarily concerned with answering the question: Does this test provide an accurate and comprehensive measure of the knowledges, skills, and attitudes presented in the course?

To build a test that has high content validity, we must:

1. Identify the overall competencies and specific behavioral outcomes to be measured.
2. Build an appropriate table of specifications (or test "blueprint").
3. Construct a test that closely mirrors the table of specifications, including individual test items that measure the levels of learning cited in the original course objectives.

Consequently, we would expect that a test developed to measure achievement in developing patient care plans would contain items measuring competence in assessment of a patient's health status, procedures for planning nursing interventions, implementation of a patient care plan, and methods for evaluating nursing interventions.

To ensure high content validity for teacher-made tests, logical analysis and careful planning using the three steps described are required.

## Criterion-related validity

The purpose of an assessment of criterion-related validity is to determine the degree of relationship between test performance and other kinds of student performance (criteria).

Criterion-related validity is of value whenever we wish to use test performance to predict future performance or to estimate current performance on some other measure. The comparison of test scores with immediate criterion performance may establish "concurrent validity"; the comparison of test scores with future criterion performance measures "predictive validity."

### Concurrent validity

Concurrent validity expresses the degree to which scores obtained on one test match current levels of behavior assessed at the same time in a second way. For example, a psychiatric outpatient center is piloting the use of a test purported to measure counseling skills. The test is given to job applicants, and on the same day the job applicants are also rated by a nursing supervisor during a counseling session. This concurrent measuring of counseling skills by use of a written test and a rating scale results in a measure of concurrent validity.

### Predictive validity

Predictive validity measures the degree to which a score on a measurement instrument can be used to predict future performance. For nursing programs, predictive validity may answer the question: Are the scores obtained with this assessment instrument useful for predicting future clinical performance?

The development of tests that have high predictive validity is one way for nursing programs to maximize efficiency (to select only those students who appear to have the interest and ability to successfully complete the program). For example, nursing instructors may wish to use the clinical performance grade to predict future job success. Consequently, the clinical performance grade is compared with the job performance evaluation at the completion of one year of employment. To the extent that the clinical performance grade had predictive validity, nursing students will be similarly ranked by both the clinical performance grade and their job performance evaluation.

### Criterion-related validity and correlation

Criterion-related validity is often called "empirical" validity or "statistical" validity because the mathematical concept of correlation is used to assess the strength of the validity. The key element in criterion-related validity is the degree of relationship between the two sets of measures: (1) the test scores, and (2) the criterion measure to be predicted or estimated. *Criterion* may be defined as "some indicator of performance that we accept as showing how successful each person has been" (Thorndike and Hagen, 1969, p. 645).

This relationship is often expressed by means of a correlation coefficient. The following discussion of correlation is designed to aid readers unfamiliar with the concept.

**Correlation coefficients.** The relationship between two variables is called a correlation. Two questions can be asked: (1) To what extent are the two variables related or similar (concurrent validity)? (2) How accurately can one variable be predicted from another (predictive validity)?

**Example:**

Does the course test average have a relationship to the laboratory performance (concurrent validity)? If the college grade point average is known, can the Nursing Board Examination score be predicted (predictive validity)?

These questions can be answered by calculating a coefficient of correlation. Numbers that are possible as coefficients of correlation range from +1.00 through 0.0 to −1.00. A coefficient of +1.00 de-

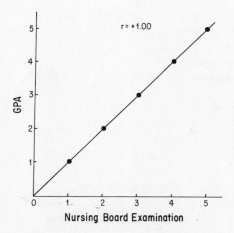

**Fig. 4-1.** Perfect positive correlation.

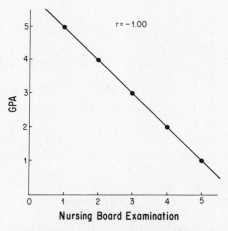

**Fig. 4-2.** Perfect negative correlation.

scribes a perfect positive correlation (as the grade point average increases, the NBE score also increases). Fig. 4-1 illustrates a perfect positive correlation plotted on a scattergram. In summary, the +1.00 correlation coefficient illustrated in Fig. 4-1 indicates that, each time one variable increases or decreases, the second variable changes in the *same* direction.

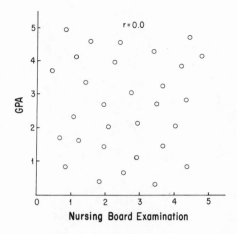

**Fig. 4-3.** No correlation.

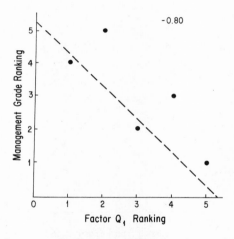

**Fig. 4-4.** Scattergram illustrating the correlation coefficient.

A coefficient of $-1.00$ describes a perfect negative correlation (as the grade point average increases, the NBE score decreases). Fig. 4-2 illustrates a perfect negative correlation plotted on a scattergram. That is, the $-1.00$ correlation coefficient illustrated in Fig. 4-2 indicates that, each time there is an increase in one variable, there is a decrease in the second variable.

A coefficient of 0.0 indicates that no relationship exists other than what might result by chance between the two variables (grade point

**Table 4-1.** Factor $Q_1$ rankings and nurse management grade rankings

| Name | Factor $Q_1$ ranking | Nursing management grade ranking |
|---|---|---|
| Paul | 1 | 4 |
| Betty | 2 | 5 |
| Tom | 3 | 2 |
| John | 4 | 3 |
| Amy | 5 | 1 |
| | $r = -0.80$ | |

average and NBE scores are unrelated). Fig. 4-3 illustrates a 0.0 correlation plotted on a scattergram.

The closer the correlation coefficient is to $+1.00$ or $-1.00$, the greater the relationship between the sets of scores. The strength of the relationship depends on the numerical value of the correlation coefficient. Therefore, $+0.90$ and $-0.90$ are equally strong; only the direction is different. The strength of the relationship is indicated by the numerical value. The direction is indicated by the sign $(+, -)$. A plus sign indicates a positive correlation, and a minus sign indicates a negative correlation.

It is extremely important to note that correlation never proves causation unless *all* related factors (age, sex, socioeconomic status, environment, and so on) are held constant or controlled in some fashion. A portion of the relationship may be the result of uncontrolled related factors. Consequently, there is no substitute for alertness and careful thought in the interpretation of such relationships.

**Example:**

The nursing faculty wish to determine if the factor $Q_1$ score on the *Sixteen Personality Factor Questionnaire* can be used to predict the final grade in nursing management. A student who scores low on the $Q_1$ factor is "conservative, respecting established ideas"; a high score represents an "experimenting person who is critical, liberal, and free thinking" (Institute for Personality and Ability Testing, 16PF, 1972, p. 17).

The hypothetical results are shown in Table 4-1, with the corresponding pattern of results shown in Fig. 4-4. In Fig. 4-4, $Q_1$ scores are shown on the horizontal axis, and management grades are shown on the vertical axis. Since the strength of the relationship is indicated by the numerical value of 0.80 and the direction of the relationship is indicated by the sign $(-)$, the relationship is strong and negative. The following conclusions can be drawn:

- As the score for factor $Q_1$ increases, the course grade in nursing management decreases. That is, as students become more experimenting, critical, and freethinking, their respective grade in nursing management decreases.
- As the score for factor $Q_1$ decreases, the respective grade in nursing management increases. As students become more conservative and respectful of established ideas, their nursing management scores may increase.

Remember, strong negative correlations are as useful in establishing predictive validity coefficients as strong positive correlations.

### Criterion measures

The real problem with establishing criterion-related validity is finding a suitable criterion measure. One of the most difficult problems that a nursing educator encounters is that of finding or developing a satisfactory measure of job success to serve as a criterion measure for test validation. Difficulties in finding satisfactory criterion measures arise from a variety of sources. For example, it is often difficult to develop an agreed-upon instrument to assess clinical nursing competence. Even when such instruments are available, they are often influenced by a variety of factors beyond the nurse's control: often the effectiveness of a nurse is not only a function of his or her ability but also of the supervision and assistance the nurse receives. Consequently, job performance ratings are influenced by many factors other than the proficiency of the person being rated.

When making decisions on the choice of a criterion measure, we should strive for a measure that is relevant, relatively free from bias, reliable, and practical. Remember, the primary limitation is the adequacy of the available criterion measures (Chase, 1974).

### Construct validity

Construct validity expresses the degree of relationship between test performance and psychological constructs or theoretical principles. We are primarily concerned with construct validity when we wish to infer from a student's test performance the student's possession of certain psychological traits or qualities. For example, instead of merely assessing a student's performance on a specific test, we may want to determine that person's self-esteem, anxiety level, or problem-solving ability. These are hypothetical qualities called "constructs." We assume the existence of these constructs so we can account for behavior in many specific situations.

There is no set procedure for determining construct validity and no single correlation coefficient. However, there are several strategies that help to establish construct validity. The first step of any strategy is to build a theory about a trait that can lead to predictions subject to empirical verification (Thorndike and Hagen, 1969). Such a theory is called a "nomological net."

The second step is to acquire evidence of construct validity in one of four ways. (Note: The overall evidence is partly rational and partly empirical [Chase, 1974]).

1. *Through predictions of group differences on a test.* Persons independently ranked high on the construct will score very differently on a test from persons independently ranked low. For example, a test might be developed to measure independence/dependence. A psychologist, familiar with identifying independent behavior, might identify a group of persons who are very independent and a group of persons who are very dependent. The test will be valid if its scores show clear independence/dependence differences between the two groups picked by the psychologist.

   Items are selected for the test from a pool of items on which the independent persons answer differently from the dependent persons. The actual content of each item is less important than the fact that the two groups responded to the item differently. For example, the question, "Do you fall asleep on your side or your back?" may seem irrelevant to a determination of independence; however, if there is a clear difference between how the two groups respond to this item, it may be used to help differentiate between the two groups.

2. *Through predictions of the effects on group differences of experimental treatments or interventions.* If a test has construct validity, conditions that will alter the construct should also affect how people score on the test. By administering our test to measure the construct independence/dependence, we can identify a group of highly dependent persons. Then, since certain behavior modification techniques should help reduce a person's dependent behavior, we can select 50% of the highly dependent persons and try to modify their behavior; we can use the other 50% as our control group. After the therapy, we can administer our test to both the treated and untreated groups. If the test has construct validity, the change in scores for the treated group should be much greater than for the untreated group.

3. *Through correlations with other tests that purport to measure the same construct.* If the test we have developed is a valid

measure of independence/dependence as defined by the theory, scores on our test should correlate with those on other tests that measure independence/dependence.

4. *Through measuring a test's internal consistency.* Additional evidence of construct validity can be found by analyzing the responses of an entire group to each separate item on the test. If our construct is a single trait, the items on the test should all be samples of the same basic behavior. That is, the proportion of people who get the first item "correct" should equal the proportion of those who get the second item "correct," and so on. This characteristic is known as "internal consistency" and can be statistically assessed, as explained in the section on test reliability.

To build a test to measure a construct, we should attempt to secure data from as many sources as possible. The more of the four techniques we use to support a claim of construct validity, the greater confidence we can have in making decisions based on the test results.

The two key elements in construct validity are:

1. Development of rational evidence based on our general knowledge of our society and the groups within it. This helps us suggest an array of group differences that seem to make sense and seem reasonable.
2. Development of empirical verification of the interpretations we propose. As indicated, this involves a variety of types of evidence.

As both rational and empirical evidence accumulate concerning the meaning of the test scores, our decisions become more useful.

### Summary

In a report of test validity, it is very important to give enough information for meaningful interpretation. For example, to report that a test has content validity is quite different from reporting that a test has high predictive validity. Much information is lost if we only report that our assessment instrument is *valid*.

### RELIABILITY

Suppose you are taking the temperature of John, age 3, in the pediatric unit. John has just been admitted; his rectal temperature is 104.5 °F. The doctor is now at the bedside and asks, "Are you sure?" He proceeds to again take John's temperature. The thermometer still records 104.5 °F. The thermometer was consistent, or reliable, in its report.

Similarly, a test is reliable to the extent that it is consistent with itself. That is, a test is reliable if it ranks the individual in essentially the same position on successive administrations.

There are three basic methods for determining test reliability. Each provides a different type of information. Consequently, the reliability coefficients obtained with the different procedures are not interchangeable. It is important that we know the specific method used before we interpret the test reliability results.

The three basic methods assess the following types of test reliability.

1. *Stability reliability*, that is, the stability of test scores over some given period of time. The test is given to the same individuals on two separate occasions. (Note: Stability reliability is also sometimes referred to as test/retest reliability.)
2. *Equivalence reliability*, that is, the consistency of test scores between different forms of the test. Two equivalent forms of a test may be developed and each form administered to the same individuals on separate occasions. (Note: Equivalent forms are also sometimes referred to as parallel forms.)
3. *Internal consistency reliability*, that is, the consistency of test scores between different parts of the test. The test may be given to a group of people and the entire group's set of scores on the first half of the test compared with the entire group's set of scores on the second half of the test.

## Stability reliability

Determination of stability reliability requires administering the same test to the same group with some intervening time interval. The length of the time interval may vary from several days to several years. However, the length of the time interval should fit the type of interpretation to be made from the results. For example, if we are interested in using test scores to group students for more efficient clinical learning, short-term reliability may be most desirable. In contrast, if we are trying to predict job success, evidence of stability over a period of years would be recommended.

To calculate the stability reliability coefficient for a test, the following procedures should be followed (Erickson and Wentling, 1976):

1. Administer the test.
2. Readminister the same test after an appropriate lapse of time.
3. Calculate the correlation coefficient.

### Example:

What is the stability reliability of the psychiatric portion of the Nursing Board Examination scores on two successive days for the same subjects?

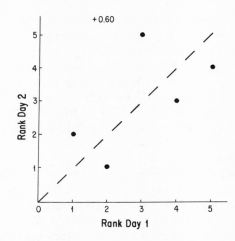

**Fig. 4-5.** Scattergram illustrating individual ranking results from two administrations of a psychiatric test.

**Table 4-2.** Individual ranking results from two administrations of a psychiatric test

| Name | Psychiatric test ranking, day 1 | Psychiatric test ranking, day 2 |
|---|---|---|
| John | 1 | 2 |
| Joy | 2 | 1 |
| Crystal | 3 | 5 |
| Arlene | 4 | 3 |
| Frank | 5 | 4 |

Table 4-2 and Fig. 4-5 illustrate the results. The stability reliability coefficient for the psychiatric portion of the NBE is found to be +0.60. Is this an acceptable reliability coefficient? There is no easy, straightforward answer. Coefficients of reliability of 0.80 and higher are regularly found for many standardized achievement tests. However, reliability coefficients for personality inventories are frequently lower (Ahmann and Glock, 1971).

The first attempt to create a test may result in a correlation between +0.50 and +0.70. Remember, a test's validity is limited by its reliability, and the teacher-made test should at least have a reliability coefficient in excess of 0.40 to be of any value. Obviously, scores from tests with low reliability coefficients must be interpreted with caution.

There are some precautions to consider in the use of stability procedures. The coefficients are influenced by day-to-day stability of the students' responses, as well as by errors inherent in the measurement procedures. For example, students may score higher on the second test administration because they learned something from taking the test the first time or because they remember how they originally responded to may items on the test. This method is not considered the most defensible for achievement tests, because of these weaknesses.

## Equivalence reliability

To determine equivalence reliability, two forms of the same test material are given to each student; consequently, two scores are available from each student, one score from form A and a second score from form B. When the two forms are administered with a significant intervening period of time, both the stability reliability and equivalence reliability can be determined. Thus, if a nursing student completes both form A and form B on January 20, only equivalence reliability can be measured; however, if the nursing student completes form A on January 20 and form B on June 20, both stability reliability and equivalence reliability can be determined.

When a significant interval has elapsed, however, three sources of variation may exist: variation arising from the test itself, variation in the student over time, and sampling variation. To ask that a test yield consistent results under these conditions is a most rigorous demand. However, many test specialists believe that the correlation between equivalent forms administered with the lapse of time represents the preferred procedure for measuring test reliability.

Truly equivalent forms of classroom tests are seldom found. Instructors usually do not construct them except for make-up tests, which theoretically should be equivalent forms but rarely are. Standardized tests, however, are often published with two equivalent forms and sometimes more.

To construct equivalent forms, the test author must have identified specific behavior objectives and developed a table of specifications based on these objectives. The author must then write two cross-sectional samples of test items that represent the same level of difficulty and the same representative sample from each cell.

### Examples of equivalent forms

OBJECTIVE: Calculate safe drug dosages for adults and children.

TEST ITEM FOR FORM A: Ms. Stern is to receive codeine sulfate gr 1/2 orally prn for pain. You have codeine sulfate 15 mg tablets available. How many tablets will you give to Ms. Stern?

TEST ITEM FOR FORM B: The order for Nisentil gr 1/4 3-4 hr is noted by the nurse. The vial is marked Nisentil 60 mg/ml. How much should she give?

OBJECTIVE: Recognize common side effects and toxic effects that may occur with each drug classification.

TEST ITEM FOR FORM A: Symptoms that may indicate cumulative effects or toxicity of digoxin is occurring include:
1. *Anorexia, nausea, vomiting, slowed pulse*
2. Abdominal pain, constipation, anorexia
3. Nausea, fast pulse, bradycardia

TEST ITEM FOR FORM B: All the following may indicate cumulative effects or toxicity of digoxin *except:*
1. Anorexia
2. Nausea
3. *Fast pulse*
4. Vomiting

## Internal consistency reliability

The assessment of internal consistency reliability is the most widely used procedure for estimating test reliability. A single test is given in a single setting. Two separate scores are derived for each student taking the test. The resulting coefficient is derived by either the Spearman-Brown Prophecy Formula or by the Kuder-Richardson procedure.

### Spearman-Brown Prophecy Formula (split-half method)

When the Spearman-Brown Prophecy Formula is used, the test is divided into two equal parts; then the scores from the two halves are correlated. When deciding how to break the test into two halves, we must make a conscious effort to balance the content and difficulty level of the two halves. Often it is suggested that we split the test into two parts by having all even numbers make up one half, whereas all odd numbers make up the other half.

Now that the test is split into equal parts, the two 50-item tests are only half as long as the original test. By using the Spearman-Brown Prophecy Formula, we can split our test and determine a correlation coefficient (Erickson and Wentling, 1976).

$$\text{Reliability of total test} = \frac{2 \times \text{reliability of } \frac{1}{2} \text{ test}}{1 \times \text{reliability of } \frac{1}{2} \text{ test}}$$

### Kuder-Richardson procedure

A second procedure for calculating test reliability is the Kuder-Richardson method. It gives a reliability estimated from item analysis data. The formula is based on the proportion of students scoring correctly on each item and the standard deviation of the test scores. The formula is cumbersome and requires a detailed item analysis. This is often the correlation coefficient that is reported for teacher-made achievement tests that are computer-scored.

Obviously, the important advantages of the internal consistency method for determining reliability have contributed to its wide use. However, it does not take into account the variation in the student from one time to the next, and it is inappropriate for speed tests. Furthermore, many standardized test manuals report only internal consistency reliability coefficients and no other reliability statistics. As informed instructors and test users, we should require commercial test builders to provide reliability estimates based on equivalent forms of the tests.

Suggestions for improving internal consistency reliability follow:
- Increase the test length. The longer the instructor-made test, the more reliable it will be. This is true if the additional items are as good as those in the shorter version and if the new test is not so long that fatigue becomes a factor.
- Replace items that are either too hard or too easy. Replacing test items that everyone answers correctly or that everyone answers incorrectly will increase the overall test reliability.
- Increase the number of alternatives or options for each test item. Just as increasing the test length will increase test reliability, increasing the number of reasonable alternatives or options for each test item will also increase test reliability.
- Write complete and clear test directions. If the instructor writes clear, complete test directions, test reliability will be increased.

**Summary**

In summary, when reliability coefficients are reported, it is very important that enough information be given for meaningful interpretation. For example, a reliability coefficient of +0.85 determined by the internal consistency split-half method is considerably different from a reliability coefficient of +0.85 determined from equivalent forms.

**PRACTICALITY**

In addition to being valid and reliable, a good test should be practical. Practicality encompasses a variety of common-sense considerations. For example, a test should be easy to administer, interpret, and score. Furthermore, it should be economical in terms of cost and time required for administration.

## Administration

A test is easy to administer if it has simple, complete directions and can be given in a reasonable amount of time. Some tests require trained personnel for administration. If these personnel are not available, it becomes impossible to ensure test validity and reliability.

## Interpretation

Ease of interpretation of the test results is another consideration in the determination of test practicality. Some tests of personality, aptitudes, and interests require trained personnel to interpret the results. Consequently, we should consider the test-related competencies of the available nursing faculty before we develop a testing protocol.

## Scoring

Ease of scoring is an equally important consideration. Some tests, such as the Rorschach projective technique for personality appraisal, require expertly trained scorers. Some group tests use time-consuming methods to determine scores for different psychological characteristics. For example, the *Sixteen Personality Factor Questionnaire* results in 16 subscores for measuring 16 personality characteristics and is very time-consuming to hand score.

## Economy

We must all consider the economy of using classroom tests or standardized tests. The cost of standardized tests to measure the same characteristic varies from publisher to publisher. The cost of creating a classroom test also varies. It is wise for us to estimate the cost of developing our own. One main cost is time.

We must also consider economy when we determine the length of our tests. Lengthy tests are costly in terms of faculty and student time. In addition, the length of a test may affect the cooperation and interest of the student being tested.

## SUMMARY

Test validity, reliability, and practicality reflect basic attributes of a test. They serve as guidelines for the nursing instructor who wishes to make informed decisions concerning teacher-made or standardized tests. Obviously, to predict human behavior and performance is hazardous at best and subject to error; however, a standardized score or a score from a well-designed instructor-made test is far superior to subjective data for this purpose. We must put into proper perspective the purposes for which our tests are designed. The current debate over these matters will in the long run be valuable if it forces us to study all the available ways for assessing nursing education.

## REFERENCES

Ahmann, J. S., and Glock, M. D.: Evaluating pupil growth, Boston, 1971, Allyn and Bacon.

Chase, C. I.: Measurement for educational evaluation, Reading, Mass., 1974, Addison-Wesley Publishing Co.

Erickson, R. C., and Wentling, T. L.: Measuring student growth; techniques and procedures for occupational education, Boston, 1976, Allyn and Bacon.

Institute for Personality and Ability Testing: Sixteen personality factor questionnaire, Champaign, Ill., 1972, The Institute.

Thorndike, R. L., and Hagen, E.: Measurement and evaluation in psychology and education, New York, 1969, John Wiley & Sons, Inc.

# 5

# A few statistics.

An essential contribution to the area of tests and measurements has been the methodology used to analyze, summarize, and interpret test data. Statistical concepts are necessary for interpreting test scores and for adequate analysis and evaluation of measuring instruments. In this chapter, the most common statistical concepts are reviewed.

Without some basic background in tests and measurements, anyone is likely to confuse "percentage-correct scores" with "percentile ranks," "percentile ranks" with "standard scores," or "mean" score with the "median" score. Without a fundamental understanding of such scores, no one can hope to accurately interpret test results.

## FREQUENCY DISTRIBUTIONS: ORGANIZATION AND PRESENTATION OF DATA

When test scores are recorded as they are gathered, the result is a mass of unorganized data. Our first step, therefore, is to organize the scores in such a way that the information becomes meaningful.

### Simple frequency distribution

The simple frequency distribution is a mechanism for ordering raw scores for ease of inspection and presentation. It provides the instructor with the following information:

- A clear indication of the range of scores. (The arrangement of test scores in a frequency distribution is usually in descending order, with the highest score placed at the top of the distribution.)
- An arrangement of scores so that the number of times a score appears (frequency) is counted.
- A rough indication of the average level of performance.

Let us suppose that the raw scores from a test on skin disorders are as follows:

18, 18, 19, 14, 16, 18, 19, 16, 17, 18, 18, 17, 16, 18,
18, 18, 18, 16, 17, 16, 19, 16

**Table 5-1.** Simple frequency distribution for skin disorder examination scores

| Score | Tally | Frequency | Cumulative frequency |
|---|---|---|---|
| 19 | ||| | 3 | 22 |
| 18 | ₦ |||| | 9 | 19 |
| 17 | ||| | 3 | 10 |
| 16 | ₦ | | 6 | 7 |
| 15 | 0 | 0 | 1 |
| 14 | | | 1 | 1 |

Construction of a simple frequency distribution would facilitate the interpretation of these test scores. Mere inspection of the raw score data rearranged as in Table 5-1 allows the instructor to make several new observations. For example, the range of scores becomes clear. The highest score is 19, and the lowest score is 14. The score most frequently achieved is 18; so 18 becomes the rough average score.

**Directions for preparing a simple frequency distribution**

1. Arrange the scores from highest to lowest with interval widths of one.
2. Using a tally column, place a slash or hash mark each time a score appears.
3. Count the number of slash or hash marks for each score, and record the number in a frequency column.
4. Decide whether to add a cumulative frequency column at the right-hand side of the frequency column. One is often included on a simple frequency distribution since it assures the instructor that each raw score has been included in the distribution. If the uppermost entry in the cumulative frequency column equals the number of test scores in the class, all scores are accounted for.
5. To complete the cumulative frequency column, begin at the bottom of the frequency column. Record the frequency in the cumulative frequency column. Then add to that cumulative frequency the frequency for the interval above. Record their sum in the cumulative frequency column. Continue this process until you have recorded all cumulative frequencies in the table. For example, the following addition provided the data for the cumulative frequency column in Table 5-1:

| Frequency | Addition process | Cumulative frequency |
|-----------|------------------|----------------------|
| 3 | 3 + 19 = | 22 |
| 9 | 9 + 10 = | 19 |
| 3 | 3 + 7 = | 10 |
| 6 | 6 + 1 = | 7 |
| 0 | 0 + 1 = | 1 |
| 1 | 1 = | 1 |

## Grouped frequency distribution

The grouped frequency distribution is a mechanism for arranging scores so that the number of times a *range* of scores appears can be counted. It sacrifices some accuracy for convenience, summarizes a large number of scores, and always has an interval width greater than one.

An instructor may group scores for the following reasons (Minium, 1970):
- When the range of scores is large, grouping facilitates interpretation of the scores.
- Grouping makes further computation easier.
- The shape or form of the score distribution is often more readily seen when scores are grouped.
- If the frequency distribution is to be represented graphically, the graph is often less confusing when scores are grouped.

The primary disadvantages to grouping scores are the following:
- Grouping yields some distortion of the data (the greater the interval width, the greater the distortion).
- It is difficult to retrieve the original scores.

Table 5-2 provides a grouped frequency distribution for the following test scores on a burn patient care examination:

42, 45, 47, 46, 38, 55, 45, 40, 39, 49, 33, 44, 45, 36, 39, 40, 46, 47, 47, 38, 46, 51, 39, 47, 39, 44, 37, 41, 36, 40, 46, 42, 35, 54, 50

## Directions for preparing a grouped frequency distribution

1. Determine the range of scores (the highest score minus the lowest score plus one). The range for the scores in Table 5-2 is 56 − 33 + 1, or 24.
2. Select an interval width. Remember, the grouping process yields some distortion of the data; therefore, the larger the interval width, the greater the distortion. An odd number is often selected for the interval width so that the midpoint will be a whole number. In Table 5-2, the interval width chosen was three.

**Table 5-2.** Grouped frequency distribution for burn patient care examination scores

| Apparent score limits | Tally | Frequency | Cumulative frequency |
|---|---|---|---|
| 54-56 | \|\| | 2 | 35 |
| 51-53 | \| | 1 | 33 |
| 48-50 | \|\| | 2 | 32 |
| 45-47 | N̸N̸ N̸N̸ \| | 11 | 30 |
| 42-44 | \|\|\|\| | 4 | 19 |
| 39-41 | N̸N̸ \|\|\| | 8 | 15 |
| 36-38 | N̸N̸ | 5 | 7 |
| 33-35 | \|\| | 2 | 2 |

3. Establish the "apparent" score limits by grouping the raw scores according to the interval width chosen. Then extend the apparent score limits 0.5 below and 0.5 above each apparent score grouping so you can establish the "real" score limits, as in the following:

| Apparent score limits | Real score limits |
|---|---|
| 54-56 | 53.5-56.5 |
| 51-53 | 50.5-53.5 |
| 48-50 | 47.5-50.5 |
| 45-47 | 44.5-47.5 |
| 42-44 | 41.5-44.5 |
| 39-41 | 38.5-41.5 |
| 36-38 | 35.5-38.5 |
| 33-35 | 32.5-35.5 |

The real score limits are used to calculate the midpoint of each interval and to retrieve data from the grouped frequency distribution.

4. Determine the midpoints of the interval, using the following procedures:
   Confirm the real interval width:

$$35.5 - 32.5 = 3.0$$

Add half of the interval width to the lower *real* limit of the interval:

$$32.5 + 1.5 = 34$$

Consequently, the midpoints for the score limits in Table 5-2 are the following:

| Apparent score limits | Real score limits | Midpoint |
|:---:|:---:|:---:|
| 54-56 | 53.5-56.5 | 55 |
| 51-53 | 50.5-53.5 | 52 |
| 48-50 | 47.5-50.5 | 49 |
| 45-47 | 44.5-47.5 | 46 |
| 42-44 | 41.5-44.5 | 43 |
| 39-41 | 38.5-41.5 | 40 |
| 36-38 | 35.5-38.5 | 37 |
| 33-35 | 32.5-35.5 | 34 |

5. Refer to the raw score distribution and tally each score, one by one, against the list of score limits.
6. Count the number of slash or hash marks for each score interval, and record the number in the frequency column.
7. Decide whether to add a cumulative frequency column to the right of the frequency column.

On occasion it may be desirable to add a percentage column to the right of the cumulative frequency column. The numbers in the percentage column are obtained by dividing the frequency $(f)$ by the total number of raw scores $(N)$ in the distribution and then multiplying by 100:

$$\frac{f}{N} \times 100 = \text{percentage}$$

where $f$ is the frequency (or times a score appears), and $N$ is the total number of raw scores. For example, two scores fall in the lowest interval (33-35) in Table 5-2. Therefore:

$$\frac{2}{35} \times 100 = 5.7\%$$

or 5.7% of all the raw scores fall in the lowest class interval. In contrast, 11 scores fall in the interval from 45 to 47, so 31.4% of all the scores fall in this interval:

$$\frac{11}{35} \times 100 = 31.4\%$$

In Table 5-3, a percentage column has been added to Table 5-2.

A cumulative percentage column may also be added to the grouped frequency distribution. A cumulative percentage indicates the number of scores that fall *at* or *below* the upper real score of the interval. Therefore, the cumulative percentage for the bottom interval

**Table 5-3.** Data from Table 5-2 with a percentage column

| Apparent<br>score<br>limits | Frequency | Cumulative<br>frequency | Percentage |
|---|---|---|---|
| 54-56 | 2 | 35 | 5.7 |
| 51-53 | 1 | 33 | 2.9 |
| 48-50 | 2 | 32 | 5.7 |
| 45-47 | 11 | 30 | 31.4 |
| 42-44 | 4 | 19 | 11.4 |
| 39-41 | 8 | 15 | 22.9 |
| 36-38 | 5 | 7 | 14.3 |
| 33-35 | 2 | 2 | 5.7 |

in Table 5-3 is 5.7%. The cumulative percentage for the next interval is equal to 5.7% + 14.3%, or 20.0%. When a percentage column is included, simple cumulative addition of the percentage column results in a cumulative percentage column. For example, the following addition of the percentage column from Table 5-3 provides a cumulative percentage column:

| Percentage | Cumulative percentage |
|---|---|
| 5.7 | 94.3 + 5.7 = 100.0 |
| 2.9 | 91.4 + 2.9 = 94.3 |
| 5.7 | 85.7 + 5.7 = 91.4 |
| 31.4 | 54.3 + 31.4 = 85.7 |
| 11.4 | 42.9 + 11.4 = 54.3 |
| 22.9 | 20.0 + 22.9 = 42.9 |
| 14.3 | 5.7 + 14.3 = 20.0 |
| 5.7 | 5.7 = 5.7 |

When no percentage column is provided, the formula for calculation of the cumulative percentage is used:

$$\frac{cf}{N} \times 100 = C\%$$

Where $cf$ is the cumulative frequency, $N$ is the total number of raw scores, and $C\%$ is the cumulative percentage.

Table 5-4 summarizes the grouped frequency distribution, illustrating the apparent score limits, real score limits, midpoint, frequency, cumulative frequency, percentage, and cumulative percentage.

**Table 5-4.** Summary of grouped frequency distribution

| Apparent score limits | Real score limits | Midpoint | Frequency | Cumulative frequency | Percentage | Cumulative percentage |
|---|---|---|---|---|---|---|
| 54-56 | 53.5-56.5 | 55 | 2 | 35 | 5.7 | 100.0 |
| 51-53 | 50.5-53.5 | 52 | 1 | 33 | 2.9 | 94.3 |
| 48-50 | 47.5-50.5 | 49 | 2 | 32 | 5.7 | 91.4 |
| 45-47 | 44.5-47.5 | 46 | 11 | 30 | 31.4 | 85.7 |
| 42-44 | 41.5-44.5 | 43 | 4 | 19 | 11.4 | 54.3 |
| 39-41 | 38.5-41.5 | 40 | 8 | 15 | 22.9 | 42.9 |
| 36-38 | 35.5-38.5 | 37 | 5 | 7 | 14.3 | 20.0 |
| 33-35 | 32.5-35.5 | 34 | 2 | 2 | 5.7 | 5.7 |

## Histograms and frequency polygons

The histogram and the frequency polygon are pictorial representations of the data presented in simple and grouped frequency distributions. Both show a pictorial relationship between scores and frequency of those scores.

### Histogram

The histogram is a bar graph. Scores from a frequency distribution can be plotted on the horizontal or $x$-axis (the abscissa) and the frequency with which each test score occurs can be plotted on the vertical or $y$-axis (the ordinate).

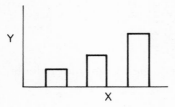

$y$ represents the frequency of each score (ordinate).
$x$ is the actual score (abscissa).

Fig. 5-1 is a histogram constructed from the data in the grouped frequency distribution for the burn patient care examination scores shown in Table 5-2. The test scores are plotted on the $x$-axis, and the frequency of each score is plotted on the $y$-axis. The histogram is constructed on the assumption that scores within an interval are evenly distributed from the lower to the upper real limits of the interval. Consequently, the upper real limit of one interval is the same as the

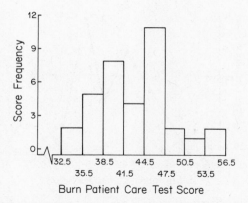

**Fig. 5-1.** Histogram: distribution of scores on burn patient care examination.

lower real limit of the next interval. As a result, there are *no* spaces between the bars of a histogram unless the frequency of an interval is equal to zero.

### Procedures for constructing a histogram

1. Mark off the score intervals along the *x*-axis. (Each interval is represented by a bar that extends from the lower to the upper real limit of the interval.)
2. Mark the score frequencies along the *y*-axis.
3. For each score interval, plot the height equivalent to the frequency of the interval already marked on the vertical axis.
4. When the frequency of an interval is zero, do not draw a bar. Leave a space for that interval.

### *Frequency polygon*

The frequency polygon is a line graph. Scores from a frequency distribution can be plotted on the horizontal or *x*-axis (the abscissa), and the frequency with which each score occurs can be plotted on the vertical or *y*-axis (the ordinate).

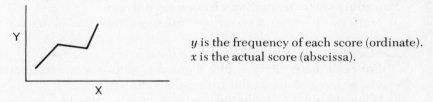

*y* is the frequency of each score (ordinate).
*x* is the actual score (abscissa).

The *midpoint* of each interval is used to plot the scores on the *x*-axis.

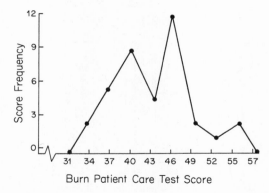

**Fig. 5-2.** Polygon: distribution of scores on burn patient care examination (interval midpoints showing).

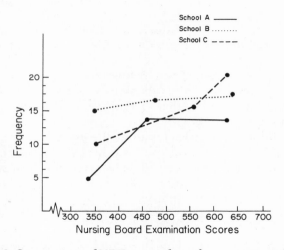

**Fig. 5-3.** Comparison of NBE scores from three nursing schools.

Fig. 5-2 is a frequency polygon constructed from the data from the grouped frequency distribution shown in Table 5-2.

**Procedures for constructing a frequency polygon**

1. Mark off the *midpoints* of the test score intervals along the *x*-axis.
2. Mark the score frequencies along the *y*-axis.
3. For each score interval, plot the point indicating the frequency of that interval above the appropriate midpoint.
4. When all points are plotted, connect each point to the next with a straight line.

5. To maintain a conventional look, anchor the frequency polygon to the horizontal axis. Midpoints are usually graphed for the intervals above and below the top and bottom intervals included in the frequency distribution, and points indicating frequencies of zero are plotted for these intervals. Consequently, when these top and bottom zero points are connected to the other points of the graph, the frequency polygon has an anchored look.

The frequency polygon is excellent for comparing scores from two or more distributions. For example, we can compare the performance of nursing students from three nursing schools on the Nursing Board Examination (NBE) by using a simple frequency polygon like that shown in Fig. 5-3. Since all three distributions can be represented on the same set of axes, comparisons are relatively easy.

## DESCRIPTIVE STATISTICS

Graphs are helpful for providing an overall view of the distribution of test scores. However, descriptive statistics provide more accurate techniques for summarizing and describing collections of data. Descriptive statistics to be discussed include measures of central tendency, position or rank, variability, and covariability.

### Central tendency

The central tendency helps the teacher answer such questions as: What is the typical Scholastic Aptitude Test (SAT) score of an entering student in the nursing program? Different measures of central tendency imply different definitions of a central, or typical, score. Common measures of central tendency are the mode, median, and mean.

#### Mode

The mode is the score that occurs most frequently in a set of scores. It is the most easily obtained measure of central tendency. In the set of scores 22, 63, 63, 80, 90, 90, 90, and 100, the mode is 90, because it occurs more often than any other score. Note: The mode is the most frequent score, 90, not the frequency of that score, which is three in this example.

**Properties of the mode.** Although the mode is easy to obtain, it is not very stable. When test scores are grouped, the mode is strongly affected by the width and location of the score intervals. For example, in the grouped score distribution in Table 5-5 the mode is 46; that is, 46 is the most frequently occurring score (46 occurs 11 times). In contrast, in Table 5-6, when these same test scores are summarized in an

**Table 5-5.** Mode from grouped frequency distribution for burn patient care examination scores

| Apparent score limits | Midpoint | Frequency |
|---|---|---|
| 54-56 | 55 | 2 |
| 51-53 | 52 | 1 |
| 48-50 | 49 | 2 |
| 45-47 | 46 | 11 |
| 42-44 | 43 | 4 |
| 39-41 | 40 | 8 |
| 36-38 | 37 | 5 |
| 33-35 | 34 | 2 |

ungrouped frequency distribution, the distributions become trimodal with the scores 39, 46, and 47 all occurring four times. Therefore, it is considered a very crude measure of typical score.

However, the mode is the preferred measure of central tendency for "nominal scale" data. Nominal scales result when observations are merely assigned to categories: for example, pass/fail, male/female, nurse/physician/medical technologist/physical therapist, or drinker/nondrinker.

Suppose you were asked to survey interest in continuing education programs for practicing nurses. You find the following: 15 nurses interested in burn care, 33 in child abuse, 11 in biofeedback and migraine headaches, and 16 in cardiac care. What measure (or measures) of central tendency would you use to report this information? Since this information is nominal-scale data, it could best be summarized by reporting the mode.

**Directions for calculating the mode for grouped data.** The mode for grouped data is the *midpoint* of the interval that contains the greatest number of scores. In Table 5-5, the mode is the midpoint of the fifth interval in the distribution. This interval contains the most frequently occurring scores. The midpoint of the interval from 45 to 47 is 46.

The mode for the grouped test scores is somewhat different from the mode of the same scores when they are ungrouped, as in Table 5-6. When the same test scores are arranged in a simple frequency distribution, the resulting distribution is trimodal, with scores of 39, 46, and 47 each appearing four times. Comparison of Tables 5-5 and 5-6 demonstrates the possible distortion of data when scores are grouped.

**Table 5-6.** Mode from simple frequency distribution for burn patient care examination scores

| Score | Tally | | Frequency | Cumulative frequency | Percentage | Cumulative percentage |
|---|---|---|---|---|---|---|
| 55 | — | | 1 | 35 | 3 | 100 |
| 54 | — | | 1 | 34 | 3 | 97 |
| 51 | — | | 1 | 33 | 3 | 94 |
| 50 | — | | 1 | 32 | 3 | 91 |
| 49 | — | | 1 | 31 | 3 | 88 |
| 47 | ≣ | —Mode— | 4 | 30 | 11 | 85 |
| 46 | ≣ | —Mode— | 4 | 26 | 11 | 74 |
| 45 | ≣ | | 3 | 22 | 8 | 63 |
| 44 | = | | 2 | 19 | 6 | 55 |
| 42 | = | | 2 | 17 | 6 | 49 |
| 41 | — | | 1 | 15 | 3 | 43 |
| 40 | ≣ | | 3 | 14 | 8 | 40 |
| 39 | ≣ | —Mode— | 4 | 11 | 11 | 32 |
| 38 | = | | 2 | 7 | 6 | 21 |
| 37 | — | | 1 | 5 | 3 | 15 |
| 36 | = | | 2 | 4 | 6 | 12 |
| 35 | — | | 1 | 2 | 3 | 6 |
| 33 | — | | 1 | 1 | 3 | 3 |

### Median

The median is the midpoint on the score scale. It has 50% of the scores below it and 50% above it. In the set of scores 4, 7, 7, 8, 10, 14, and 17, the median is 8, since three scores occur below 8 and three above 8. In the set of scores 1, 4, 5, 9, 11, and 14, the median is halfway between 5 and 9; consequently, 7 is the median.

**Properties of the median.** Although the median is sensitive to the exact number of scores above and below it, it is less sensitive than the mean to the presence of a few extreme scores. For example, in the set of scores 5, 6, 7, 8, and 50, the median is 7, with two scores above it and two scores below it; the mean is 15.2. The top score, 50, is an extreme score when compared with the remaining four scores. Whereas the score of 50 strongly affects the mean score, it is just another score above the median.

Sometimes an instructor encounters a test score distribution that is reasonably regular except for a few extreme scores. If there is concern that these extreme scores will carry undue weight in determining the mean, a possible solution is to calculate and also report the median score. Similarly, in asymmetrical or skewed distributions, the median is often a preferred measure of typical score.

The following example further illustrates the use of the median as a preferred measure of central tendency. Below are salaries for professional personnel employed in a small, family-practice clinic:

| | |
|---|---|
| Chief physician | $200,000 |
| Physician | 50,000 |
| Physician | 35,000 |
| Nurse supervisors (2) | 20,000 |
| | 15,000 |
| Nurses (10) | 10,000 |
| | 10,000 |
| | 10,000  — Median salary |
| | 10,000 |
| | 10,000 |
| | 10,000 |
| | 10,000 |
| | 10,000 |
| | 10,000 |
| | 10,000 |
| TOTAL PAYROLL | $420,000 |

The mean salary for these 15 professionals is $28,000. However, it would be misleading to report that the average person in the clinic earns $28,000. Reporting the median salary of $10,000 would be a more correct description of the typical salary.

**Table 5-7.** Median from grouped frequency distribution for burn patient care examination scores

| Apparent score limits | Real score limits | Frequency | Cumulative frequency | |
|---|---|---|---|---|
| 54-56 | 53.5-56.5 | 2 | 35 | |
| 51-53 | 50.5-53.5 | 1 | 33 | |
| 48-50 | 47.5-50.5 | 2 | 32 | |
| 45-47 | 44.5-47.5 | 11 | 30 | |
| 42-44 | 41.5-44.5 — Median interval — 4 | | 19 | |
| 39-41 | 38.5-41.5 | 8 | 15 | — Sum of frequencies |
| 36-38 | 35.5-38.5 | 5 | 7 | up to, but *not* |
| 33-35 | 32.5-35.5 | 2 | 2 | including, median interval |

**Directions for calculating the median for grouped data.** When scores have been arranged in a grouped frequency distribution, the median is still the middle score. However, calculation of the median is more complex for grouped score distributions. Table 5-7 contains the data needed to compute the *median* from grouped test scores.

Actual computational steps to determine the median for grouped data follow:

| Sequence of steps | Example |
|---|---|
| 1. To determine the median or middle score, divide the total number of test scores by 2. | In Table 5-7, the total number of scores is 35; thus, 35 ÷ 2 = 17.5. |
| 2. Beginning with the lowest interval in the cumulative frequency column, determine the interval that contains the 17.5th score. | The fourth interval, 42 to 44, contains the 17.5th score. This is the "median interval." |
| 3. Determine the real lower limit of the median interval. | The real lower limit of the median interval is 41.5. The interval width is 3.0. The sum of the frequencies up to the median interval is 15. |
| 4. Determine the interval width. | |
| 5. Determine the sum of the frequencies up to, but *not* including, the median interval. | |
| 6. Determine the frequency of the median interval. | The frequency of the median interval is 4. |
| 7. Apply the following formula to calculate the median: | |

| Sequence of steps | Example |
|---|---|

$$\text{Median} = LL + i\frac{(N/2) - cf}{fm}$$

$$41.5 + 3\frac{(35/2) - 15}{4} =$$

$$41.5 + 3\ (0.62) = 43.36$$

where *LL* is the real lower limit of the median interval, *i* is the interval width, *N* is the total number of raw scores, *cf* is the sum of the frequencies up to, but *not* including, the median interval, and *fm* is the frequency of the median interval.

The median for the grouped data is 43.36.

### Mean

The mean is often referred to as the "average," but this term should not be used in a discussion of statistical concepts, since the mode and median are also averages in the sense of being indicators of central tendency. The mean is the *arithmetic* average, that is, the score found by summing all raw scores and dividing by the total number of raw scores. Algebraically, this means:

$$\bar{x} = \frac{\Sigma x}{N}$$

where $\bar{x}$ is the mean, $\Sigma$ indicates the summation of, $x$ is the raw score, and $N$ is the total number of scores. For example, in the set of scores 4, 9, 10, 8, and 9, the mean is calculated in the following way:

$$\frac{(4 + 9 + 10 + 8 + 9)}{5} = \frac{40}{5} = 8.0$$

**Properties of the mean.** The mean, unlike any other measure of central tendency, is responsive to the exact position of each test score. If any test score is increased or decreased, the value of the mean will reflect the change (Minium, 1970). The mean may be thought of as the balance point of the distribution, that is, the score point at which the distribution balances. Fig. 5-4 illustrates this concept (Minium, 1970). Imagine a seesaw consisting of a fulcrum (balance point) with the scores of a distribution spread along the board. The mean corresponds to the position of the fulcrum, that is, the point at which the distribution balances.

There is also an algebraic way of stating that the mean is the balance point: the sum of the deviations from the mean equals zero

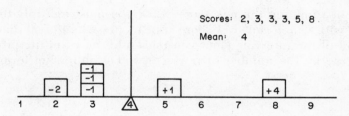

**Fig. 5-4.** Mean: score point where the distribution balances.

**Table 5-8.** Mean from grouped frequency distribution for burn
patient care examination scores

| Apparent score limits | Midpoint | Frequency | *f(M)* (midpoint × frequency) |
|---|---|---|---|
| 54-56 | 55 | 2 | 110 |
| 51-53 | 52 | 1 | 52 |
| 48-50 | 49 | 2 | 98 |
| 45-47 | 46 | 11 | 506 |
| 42-44 | 43 | 4 | 172 |
| 39-41 | 40 | 8 | 320 |
| 36-38 | 37 | 5 | 185 |
| 33-35 | 34 | 2 | 68 |
| | | | 1,511 |

$(\Sigma(x - \bar{x}) = 0)$. That is, when each score is expressed in terms of how
far it deviates from the mean, the sum equals zero. For example, for
the scores shown in Fig. 5-4, we have the following:

| Score | Mean | Score − mean |
|---|---|---|
| 8 | 4 | $8 - 4 = +4$ |
| 2 | 4 | $2 - 4 = -2$ |
| 3 | 4 | $3 - 4 = -1$ |
| 3 | 4 | $3 - 4 = -1$ |
| 3 | 4 | $3 - 4 = -1$ |
| 5 | 4 | $5 - 4 = +1$ |
| | | $\Sigma(x - \bar{x}) = 0$ |

When further statistical computation is required, the mean is the
most useful measure of central tendency.

**Directions for calculating the mean from grouped data.** The procedure for calculating the mean from grouped data is similar to that
used in computing the mean from a simple distribution. However,

instead of summing the raw scores ($\Sigma x$), you must multiply the frequency with which *each* raw score appears in each interval times the midpoint of the interval. Then you must add the resulting products and divide by the number of raw scores. The following formula is used:

$$\bar{x} = \frac{\Sigma f(M)}{N}$$

where $\bar{x}$ is the mean, $\Sigma$ indicates the summation of, $f$ is the frequency of the interval, $M$ is the midpoint of the interval, and $N$ is the total number of raw test scores. Table 5-8 gives the data needed to compute the mean from grouped test scores.

Actual computational steps to determine the mean from grouped data follow:

| Sequence of steps | Example |
|---|---|
| 1. Determine the score limits. | In Table 5-8, the score limits are 33 to 35, 36 to 38, and so forth. |
| 2. Determine the midpoint of each score interval. | Midpoints are 34, 37, and so on. |
| 3. Determine the frequency for each score interval. | The frequencies are 2, 5, 8, 4, 11, 2, 1, and 2. |
| 4. For each score interval, multiply the frequency by the midpoint of the interval in which it appears. | In the interval from 33 to 35, for example, the midpoint is 34 and there are two scores contained in this interval; therefore, $2 \times 34 = 68$. |
| 5. Sum each value in the midpoint $\times$ frequency column. | Thus, from Table 5-8, $110 + 52 + 98 + 506 + 172 + 320 + 185 + 68 = 1,511$. |
| 6. Divide the total for the midpoint $\times$ frequency column by the total number of raw test scores. | Thus, $1,511 \div 35 = 43.17$. |

The mean, thus computed, differs slightly from the mean of 42.1 that can be calculated from the ungrouped score distribution shown in Table 5-6, as follows:

$$\bar{x} = \frac{\Sigma x}{N}$$

$$\bar{x} = \frac{1,472}{35} = 42.1$$

This finding further supports the contention that grouping test scores tends to slightly distort the data.

### Summary

Each measure of central tendency has characteristics that make it uniquely valuable. The mode is the easiest to determine; often it can be found at a glance. Also, in a large, normal distribution of scores, the mode is a fairly stable measure of the center of the distribution. The median is especially useful as a measure of central tendency when distributions are skewed, for example, when all the scores are either very high or very low. Using the median when the distribution is skewed is preferred in situations in which the experimental question is concerned with the typical scores, because the median is closest to the typical score. The mean is affected by the individual values of all the scores in a set of data (whereas the median and the mode may not be). The mean is especially affected by extreme scores, that is, by scores that are far from the center of the group of scores.

Of the three measures of central tendency, the mean is the most commonly used; many advanced statistical procedures are built on or related to it. In addition, the mean is preferred to express the central tendency of a normal distribution and is necessary when interest is centered on the numerical value of all scores.

## Variability

A measure of dispersion (or variability) will help to determine the extent to which the scores in a set scatter about or cluster together. Different measures of dispersion imply different definitions of variability. The most common measures of dispersion are range, variance, and standard deviation.

### Range

The range is the difference between the highest score and the lowest score, plus one. In the set of scores 22, 63, 63, 80, and 100, the range is 79. Note: The major limitation of the range is that, since it is based on only two scores, it fails to reflect scores between the extremes.

As a measure of variability, range is a distance, in contrast to a measure of central tendency, which is a point on a score scale. The range may be determined in two ways (Gellman, 1973):

1. By subtracting the lowest score from the highest score and adding one.
2. By subtracting the lower real limit of the lowest score from the upper real limit of the highest score.

**Table 5-9.** Distribution of surgical nursing test scores

| Score | Frequency |
|-------|-----------|
| 351 | 1 |
| 352 | 2 |
| 354 | 3 |
| 355 | 0 |
| 356 | 9 |
| 357 | 3 |
| 358 | 2 |

**Table 5-10.** Number of hours spent in obstetric clinic per week

| Week | Clinic hours | |
|------|-------|-----|
| | Julie | Amy |
| 1 | 2 | 2 |
| 2 | 3 | 8 |
| 3 | 4 | 10 |
| 4 | 5 | 15 |
| 5 | 6 | 25 |

If we used each of these methods to compute the range of the distribution shown in Table 5-9, our results would be the following:

Range = highest score − lowest score + 1
Range = 358 − 351 + 1 = 7 + 1 = 8
Range = upper real limit
        of highest score − lower real limit
        of lowest score
Range = 358.5 − 350.5 = 8

**Properties of the range.** Since the range is merely a measure of the number of raw score points within a distribution, it is affected by one or more extreme scores. Obviously, this makes interpretation of the range rather tenuous. It is of value only as a rough indicator of variability. In addition, since it is determined by the two most extreme score, it is very unstable.

Table 5-10 shows the number of clinic hours Amy and Julie have spent in obstetric nursing per week over a five-week period. If we compare the range of hours each spent in the clinic, we find the following:

**Table 5-11.** Distribution of microbiology test scores

| Apparent score limits | Real score limits | Class A | Class B |
|---|---|---|---|
| 54-56 | 53.5-56.5 | 2 | 2 |
| 51-53 | 50.5-53.5 | 0 | 1 |
| 48-50 | 47.5-50.5 | 0 | 2 |
| 45-47 | 44.5-47.5 | 31 | 11 |
| 42-44 | 41.5-44.5 | 0 | 4 |
| 39-41 | 38.5-41.5 | 0 | 8 |
| 36-38 | 35.5-38.5 | 0 | 5 |
| 33-35 | 32.5-35.5 | 2 | 2 |

- Julie's hours spent in the clinic ranged from 2 to 6 per week (range = 6 − 2 + 1 = 5).
- Amy's hours spent in the clinic ranged from 2 to 25 per week (range = 25 − 2 + 1 = 24).

The number of hours Amy spent shows more variability, since the range of her hourly distribution is greater.

Table 5-11 illustrates the test scores for two sections of microbiology. Each section contains 35 students. The range is equal for both classes (range = 24.0). This would seem to indicate that the variability was equal for both classes. However, visual inspection of the grades and common sense show a greater variability of test scores in class B. Consequently, in this case the range does not accurately describe the variability of the test scores *within* the distribution.

### Variance

Variance and the standard deviation are closely related. The variance is a measure of the *spread* of scores from the center of the distribution. It is a special kind of mean, a mean that is the sum of the squared deviations from the mean of the distribution, divided by the total number of raw scores.

**Directions for calculating the variance.** To calculate the variance, compute the difference between each score and the mean, square the difference, sum these values, and divide by the total number of raw scores, as in the following formula:

$$s^2 = \frac{\Sigma(x - \bar{x})^2}{N}$$

where $s^2$ is the variance, $\Sigma$ indicates the summation of, $x$ is the raw score, $\bar{x}$ is the mean, and $N$ is the total number of raw scores. For example, for the set 1, 1, 3, 5, and 5, the mean and variance are computed as follows:

| Score | Score − mean | (Score − mean)² |
|-------|--------------|------------------|
| 1 | 1 − 3 = −2 | 4 |
| 1 | 1 − 3 = −2 | 4 |
| 3 | 3 − 3 = 0 | 0 |
| 5 | 5 − 3 = +2 | 4 |
| 5 | 5 − 3 = +2 | 4 |
| 15 | | 16 |

$$\bar{x} = \frac{\Sigma x}{N} = \frac{15}{5} = 3.0$$

$$s^2 = \frac{\Sigma(x - \bar{x})^2}{N} - \frac{16}{5} = 3.2$$

### Standard deviation

The standard deviation is the positive square root of the variance. It can also be defined as an average of the spread of the scores from the center of the distribution. It is preferred to variance as a descriptive tool because it is expressed in original raw score units, whereas variance is expressed in square units. Consequently, the standard deviation can be graphically represented, whereas variance cannot. The standard deviation is a distance on the score scale; the variance is a squared distance.

**Properties of the standard deviation.** Like the mean, the standard deviation is sensitive to the exact position of every score in the distribution. If a test score is added that is far away from the mean, the standard deviation will increase. In contrast, if a score is added that is very close to the mean, the standard deviation will decrease.

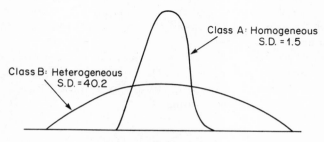

**Fig. 5-5.** Variability between Class A and Class B.

The numerical value of the standard deviation indicates the spread of the set of test scores from the mean. For example, if an instructor gives the same examination to two classes, a standard deviation of 1.5 in class A indicates that most of the scores cluster tightly around the mean; in contrast, a standard deviation of 40.2 in class B indicates that most of the scores are spread away from the mean. That is, class A is relatively homogeneous; class B is quite heterogeneous. Fig. 5-5 is a visual representation of the variability between two such classes.

The total number of test scores in a distribution does not affect the numerical value of the standard deviation. For example, a standard deviation of 2.2 could be the measure of variability for 30 test scores or for 500 test scores.

The standard deviation is independent from the mean. The size of the mean has no influence on the size of the standard deviation.

Widely accepted as the best measure of variability, the standard deviation provides the theoretical and conceptual basis for calculating and interpreting standard scores discussed in this chapter.

**Directions for calculating the standard deviation.** Computing the standard deviation requires one additional step beyond computation of the variance. Once the variance has been computed, its positive square root is the standard deviation:

$$s = \sqrt{\frac{\Sigma(x - \bar{x})^2}{N}}$$

where $s$ is the standard deviation, $\Sigma$ indicates the summation of, $x$ is the raw score, $\bar{x}$ is the mean, $N$ is the total number of raw scores, and $\sqrt{\phantom{x}}$ indicates square root. For example, the standard deviation for the set 1, 1, 3, 5, and 5 is computed in the following way:

$$s = \sqrt{\frac{\Sigma(x - \bar{x})^2}{N}} = \sqrt{\frac{16}{5}} = \sqrt{3.2} = 1.79$$

**Table 5-12.** Standard deviation

| Score | Mean | Score − mean | (Score − mean)² |
|-------|------|--------------|-----------------|
| 8 | 6 | 8 − 6 = +2 | 4 |
| 5 | 6 | 5 − 6 = −1 | 1 |
| 2 | 6 | 2 − 6 = −4 | 16 |
| 11 | 6 | 11 − 6 = +5 | 25 |
| 3 | 6 | 3 − 6 = −3 | 9 |
| 7 | 6 | 7 − 6 = +1 | 1 |
| 36 | | | 56 |

The following example indicates how to calculate the standard deviation for the raw scores from Table 5-12:

| Sequence of steps | Example |
|---|---|
| 1. Compute the mean. | In Table 5-12, the mean equals 6. |
| 2. Subtract the mean from each raw score in the distribution. | Thus, $8 - 6 = +2$; $5 - 6 = -1$; $2 - 6 = -4$; and so on. |
| 3. Square each difference or deviation score. | When negative numbers are squared, the sign becomes positive; therefore, $(-1)^2 = +1$, $(-4)^2 = +16$. |
| 4. Sum the squared difference scores. | The sum of the squared difference scores equals 56. |
| 5. Divide this sum by the total number of scores in the distribution. | Thus 56 is divided by the total number of scores in the distribution: $56 \div 6 = 9.33$. |
| 6. Compute the square root. | The square root of 9.33 is 3.05. Thus, 3.05 is the standard deviation. |

## Summary

Measures of central tendency describe only the central points of a distribution. They tell nothing about what happens away from the center of distribution. The *amount* that a distribution spreads from the center is also important and is measured by its variability or dispersion. For example, a nursing instructor with two classes of three students each may decide to rely on mathematics test scores to determine whether to use the same instructional procedures and materials to teach drug dosages to both classes. Following are the test scores, mean, median, range, and standard deviation for class A and class B:

| Class A | | Class B | |
|---|---|---|---|
| Ann | 101 | Eve | 150 |
| Charles | 100 | Fred | 100 |
| Donald | 99 | Gloria | 50 |
| Mean | 100 | Mean | 100 |
| Median | 100 | Median | 100 |
| Range | 2 | Range | 100 |
| Standard deviation | 0.81 | Standard deviation | 40.8 |

The instructor who bases decisions on measures of central tendency alone would probably decide to teach both classes in the same way, since both class A and class B have test means and medians of 100. However, the instructor who inspects the measures of variability (the range and the standard deviation) will realize how disastrous considering central tendency only would be. Scores in class B have considerably greater variability than scores in class A. By reviewing both

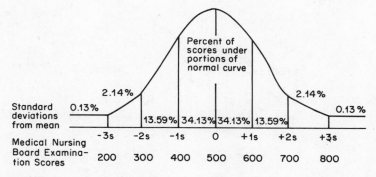

**Fig. 5-6.** Relationship of standard deviation to the normal curve for NBE medical nursing examination scores.

central tendency and variability, the instructor may decide to continue lecturing to class A but to enrich class B with media aids such as programmed texts and computer-assisted instruction. The instructor may also decide to provide remedial help for Gloria and enrichment for Eve.

### The normal curve

The relationship of standard deviation to the normal curve is important in the interpretation of test scores that are normally distributed. The normal curve is a mathematical model that expresses the relationship between the standard deviation and the proportion of cases. The same proportion of cases will always be found within the same standard deviation units.

By referring to the relationship of standard deviation to normal curve in Fig. 5-6, you can see that the following statements are true:
- Deviations below the mean are preceded by a minus sign, those above the mean by a plus sign.
- About 68% of the population falls between −1 standard deviation and +1 standard deviation (68.26% of the population's Nursing Board Examination medical nursing scores fall between 400 and 600).
- About 34% of the scores fall within −1 standard deviation from the mean or within +1 standard deviation from the mean (34.13% of the population have scores between 500 and 600, and 34.13% have scores between 400 and 500).
- About 95% of the population falls between −2 standard deviations and +2 standard deviations from the mean (95.44% of the population's scores fall between 300 and 700).
- About 99% of the population falls between −3 standard devia-

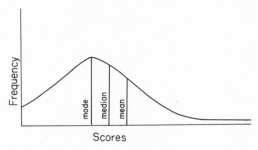

**Fig. 5-7.** Positively skewed curve.

tions and +3 standard deviations from the mean (99.74% of the population's scores fall between 200 and 800).

**Properties of normal curves.** All normal curves are symmetrical about the mean. That is, the right half of the curve is a mirror image of the left half of the curve. Since the curve is symmetrical, the mean, mode, and median are equal. The limits of the curve are plus and minus infinity. Thus, the extreme ends of the curve never touch the baseline. The normal curve is unimodal. The curve will have a standard deviation equal to one when the values are expressed in terms of $z$ values. Note: Before you can use the standard normal distribution, test scores must be transformed into a "standard normal variable."

### Skewed distributions

Often, test score distributions do not take the form of a normal distribution. That is, the score distributions are skewed. If a test elicits many low scores, a positively skewed curve, as shown in Fig. 5-7, will result. When a set of scores is positively skewed, the mode, median, and mean are no longer equal. In almost any unimodal, positively skewed distribution, we find the relationships shown in Fig. 5-7:

- The *mode* is on the left, with the lowest score value, but as its definition dictates, with the highest frequency value.
- The *median* is in the middle.
- The *mean* is on the right, with the highest numerical scores. A little thought will tell you why. In a positively skewed distribution, the hump is on the left; therefore, the mode must be a low value. The tail, with its *extreme* values, is on the right. Consequently, the mean, which is affected by *every* score, is pulled to the right by the extreme scores and is a high value.

In contrast, if a test elicits many high scores, a negatively skewed curve, as shown in Fig. 5-8, will result. Again, if a set of scores is negatively skewed, the mode, median, and mean are no longer equal. In

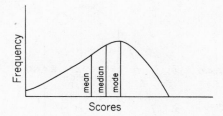

**Fig. 5-8.** Negatively skewed curve.

almost any unimodal, negatively skewed curve, we find the relation-
ships illustrated in Fig. 5-8:
- The *mode* is on the right, with the highest score value.
- The *median* again is in the middle.
- The mean is pulled to the left, with the lowest numerical scores,
  because it is affected by the extreme scores.

Note: For both curves (negatively and positively skewed), the three
measures of central tendency are found in alphabetical order, starting
from the tail of the curve.

The relationship between the mean and median in skewed curves
is clear enough that some writers recommend calculating an index of
skewness based on the difference between their values (Minium,
1970):

$$\text{Mean} - \text{median} = \text{skewness index}$$

- If the *mean* is greater than the median, the index is positive, indicating positive skewness.

For example, if the mean equals 15 and the median equals 12, by
applying the skewness index we get the following:

$$15 - 12 = +3$$

The resulting +3 suggests the curve, or test score distribution, is
positively skewed.

- If the *median* is greater than the mean, the index is negative,
  indicating negative skewness.

For example, if the mean equals 35 and the median equals 45, by
applying the skewness index we get the following:

$$35 - 45 = -10$$

The resulting −10 suggests the curve, or test score distribution,
is negatively skewed.

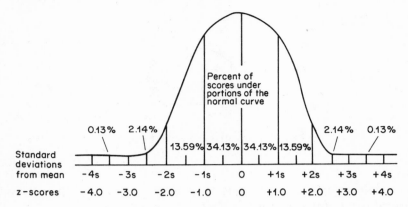

**Fig. 5-9.** Relationship of z-scores to the normal curve.

## Standard scores

Standard scores have properties that make them valuable. For example, standard scores (1) are based on the mean and standard deviation of the distribution, (2) retain the shape of the raw score distribution, (3) can be treated mathematically, and (4) permit between- and within-group comparisons.

Three standard scores are discussed in this section; z-scores, T-scores, and NBE scores.

### The z-score

The basic standard score is a z-score. It tells how many standard deviations any specified raw score is above or below the mean of the distribution. The z-score compares the performance of an individual with the performance of other individuals on the same test. It allows for comparison of students among test distributions. Its distribution has the same form as the original raw score distribution. We can average z-scores, just as we can raw scores.

The following statements are true for all z-scores:

- The mean of a distribution of z-scores is always zero, and the standard deviation is always one.
- A z-score of zero corresponds to a raw score that lies exactly at the mean.
- A *negative* z-score indicates that the raw score lies *below* the mean.
- A *positive* z-score indicates that the raw score lies *above* the mean.
- The *greater* the numerical value of a z-score, the farther the z-score lies from the mean.

**Table 5-13.** z-Scores on genetics examination*

| Student | Score | Mean | Raw score – mean | z-Score |
|---------|-------|------|------------------|---------|
| Arlene | 25 | 18 | 7 | +1.63 |
| Irene | 23 | 18 | 5 | +1.16 |
| Monica | 22 | 18 | 4 | +0.93 |
| Thomas | 20 | 18 | 2 | +0.47 |
| Paula | 18 | 18 | 0 | 0 |
| Stephanie | 17 | 18 | −1 | −0.23 |
| Erica | 16 | 18 | −2 | −0.47 |
| Pat | 15 | 18 | −3 | −0.70 |
| Karen | 14 | 18 | −4 | −0.93 |
| Joanne | 10 | 18 | −8 | −1.86 |

- The shape of the distribution is the same as the shape of the original raw score data. Thus, if the original distribution is positively skewed, the z-score equivalents will form a distribution that is positively skewed.

Fig. 5-9 illustrates the relationship of z-scores to the normal curve.

**Directions for computing the z-score.** The z-score is calculated from the raw scores in the following manner:

$$z = \frac{x - \bar{x}}{\sigma}$$

where $z$ is the z-score, $x$ is the raw score, $\bar{x}$ is the mean, and $\sigma$ is the standard deviation.

| Sequence of steps | Example |
|---|---|
| 1. Calculate the mean. | From Table 5-13, the mean is 18. |
| 2. Subtract the mean from each raw score to obtain a distance from the mean score. | The distance score for Arlene is $25 - 18 = +7$. |
| 3. Calculate the standard deviation. | The standard deviation is: $\sqrt{\frac{188}{10}} = \sqrt{18.8} = 4.3$ |
| 4. Divide the distance from the mean score by the standard deviation to obtain the z-score. | Thus, 7 divided by 4.3 is equal to a z-score of +1.63. |

**Interpreting the z-score.** To facilitate the interpretation of z-scores

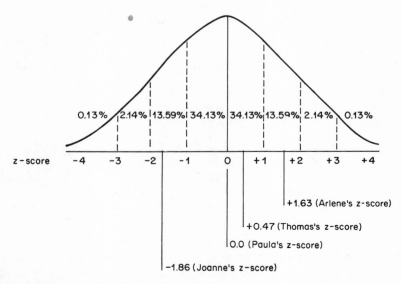

**Fig. 5-10.** Relationship of selected students' z-scores to the normal curve for genetics examination scores.

calculated for Table 5-13, the following discussion of the z-scores for Arlene, Thomas, Paula, and Joanne is presented:

| Student | z-Score | Discussion |
|---------|---------|------------|
| Arlene | +1.63 | Arlene's z-score is preceded by a plus sign. This means her score is above the mean. The greater the numerical value of the z-score, the farther the z-score lies from the mean. Thus, Arlene's score lies considerably above the mean. Its position is illustrated in Fig. 5-10. |
| Thomas | +0.47 | Thomas' z-score is preceded by a plus sign; thus, it is above the mean. Since the numerical value is low, we know the score lies near the mean. Its position is illustrated in Fig. 5-10. |
| Paula | 0.0 | Paula's z-score lies exactly at the mean. Its position is illustrated in Fig. 5-10. |
| Joanne | −1.86 | Joanne's z-score is preceded by a minus sign; thus, it is below the mean. Since the numerical value is high and negative, the score lies considerably below the mean. Its position is plotted in Fig. 5-10. |

To illustrate that z-scores, or standard scores, allow for comparison of students among different test distributions, a specific example is useful. Achievement tests in mathematics, biology, and chemistry were given to a large class of nursing students, with the following results:

|  | Mathematics | Biology | Chemistry |
|---|---|---|---|
| Anne | 82 | 74 | 83 |
| Mean | 82 | 77 | 86 |
| Standard deviation | 6.5 | 8.7 | 5.6 |

In what subject did Anne do best? To answer the question, first calculate Anne's $z$-score for each achievement test:

**Mathematics**
$$z = \frac{x - \bar{x}}{\sigma} = \frac{82 - 82}{6.5} = 0.0$$

**Biology**
$$z = \frac{x - \bar{x}}{\sigma} = \frac{74 - 77}{8.7} = \frac{-3.0}{8.7} = -0.34$$

**Chemistry**
$$z = \frac{x - \bar{x}}{\sigma} = \frac{83 - 86}{5.6} = \frac{-3.0}{5.6} = -0.54$$

By merely considering Anne's raw scores (82 in mathematics, 74 in biology, and 83 in chemistry), we might conclude that Anne did best in chemistry. However, by converting the raw scores to standard scores (in this case, $z$-scores), it becomes clear that Anne actually did her poorest in chemistry and best in math.

Although $z$-scores have many advantages (they do not distort differences, they show the distance of each score from the mean, and they can be averaged), they are difficult to work with because of the negative values and the decimal points. By multiplying each $z$-score by a constant, we can eliminate the decimal point. By adding a constant value, we can eliminate the negative sign. These mathematical procedures are followed for the standard scores discussed in the sections on $T$-scores and NBE scores.

### T-score

The $T$-score is a commonly used standard score. It can be obtained by multiplying the $z$-score by ten, then adding 50. The following statements are always true for $T$-scores:
- The mean is equal to 50.
- The standard deviation is equal to ten.
- The shape of the distribution is the same as the shape in the original raw score data. Thus, if the original distribution is positively

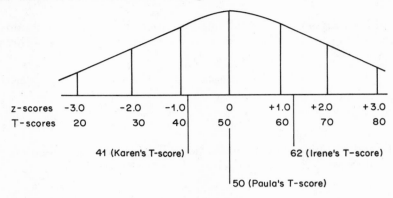

| z-scores | -3.0 | | -2.0 | -1.0 | 0 | +1.0 | +2.0 | +3.0 |
| T-scores | 20 | | 30 | 40 | 50 | 60 | 70 | 80 |

41 (Karen's T-score)                                        62 (Irene's T-score)

50 (Paula's T-score)

**Fig. 5-11.** Relationship of $z$-scores and $T$-scores to the normal curve for genetics examination scores.

skewed, the $T$-score equivalents will form a distribution that is positively skewed.

Fig. 5-11 illustrates the relationship of $z$-scores and $T$-scores, given a normal distribution.

**Directions for computing the T-score.** The $T$-score is calculated from the raw scores in the following manner:

$$T = 10\left(\frac{x - \bar{x}}{\sigma}\right) + 50$$

where $T$ is the $T$-score, $x$ is the raw score, $\bar{x}$ is the mean, and $\sigma$ is the standard deviation.

| Sequence of steps | Example |
|---|---|
| 1. Calculate the $z$-score. | In Table 5-14, the $z$-score is given for each raw score value. |
| 2. Multiply the $z$-score by 10. | For Arlene the calculation is $+1.63 \times 10 = 16.3$. |
| 3. Add 50. | Thus, $16.3 + 50 = 66.3$. Arlene's $T$-score is rounded off to 66. |

**Interpreting the T-score.** To facilitate the interpretation of $T$-scores calculated for Table 5-14, the following discussion of Irene's, Paula's, and Karen's scores is presented.

| Student | T-score | Discussion |
|---|---|---|
| Irene | 62 | Since the mean for the $T$-score is 50, Irene's score is above the mean. In addition, since the standard deviation for a $T$-score is equal to 10, Irene's score is a little higher than 1 standard deviation above the mean. Its position is illustrated in Fig. 5-11. |

**Table 5-14.** *T*-scores on genetics examination

| Student | Score | Mean | Raw score − mean | *z*-Score | *T*-score |
|---|---|---|---|---|---|
| Arlene | 25 | 18 | 7 | +1.63 | 66 |
| Irene | 23 | 18 | 5 | +1.16 | 62 |
| Monica | 22 | 18 | 4 | +0.93 | 59 |
| Thomas | 20 | 18 | 2 | +0.47 | 55 |
| Paula | 18 | 18 | 0 | 0 | 50 |
| Stephanie | 17 | 18 | −1 | −0.23 | 48 |
| Erica | 16 | 18 | −2 | −0.47 | 45 |
| Pat | 15 | 18 | −3 | −0.70 | 43 |
| Karen | 14 | 18 | −4 | −0.93 | 41 |
| Joanne | 10 | 18 | −8 | −1.86 | 31 |

| Student | T-score | Discussion |
|---------|---------|------------|
| Paula | 50 | Paula's T-score lies exactly at the mean. Its position is illustrated in Fig. 5-11. |
| Karen | 41 | Karen's T-score is below 50; thus, it is below the mean. In fact, it is almost one full standard deviation below the mean. Its position is illustrated in Fig. 5-11. |

### Nursing Board Examination scores

The Nursing Board Examination (NBE) score is a third type of standard score. It is similar to the z-score and T-score, except that it has a mean of 500 and a standard deviation of 100. Each separate subtest of the NBE (medical nursing, surgical nursing, obstetric nursing, nursing of children, and psychiatric nursing) is scored and considered separately.

Fig. 5-12 shows the relationship of NBE scores to z-scores, given a normal distribution.

**Directions for computing the Nursing Board Examination score.** The NBE score is calculated from the raw scores in the following manner:

$$\text{NBE score} = 100\left(\frac{x - \bar{x}}{\sigma}\right) + 500$$

where NBE score is the Nursing Board Examination score, $x$ is the raw score, $\bar{x}$ is the mean, and $\sigma$ is the standard deviation.

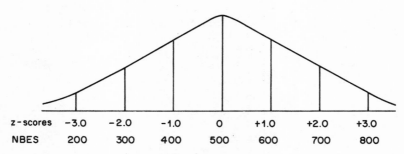

| z-scores | -3.0 | -2.0 | -1.0 | 0 | +1.0 | +2.0 | +3.0 |
|----------|------|------|------|---|------|------|------|
| NBES | 200 | 300 | 400 | 500 | 600 | 700 | 800 |

**Fig. 5-12.** Relationship of selected NBE scores to the normal curve.

**Table 5-15.** Conversion of raw scores to NBE scores

| Student | Subtest | Raw score | Mean | Raw score − mean | z-Score | NBE score |
|---------|---------|-----------|------|------------------|---------|-----------|
| Arlene | Medical nursing | 40 | 35 | +5 | +1.25 | 625 |
| Irene | Surgical nursing | 39 | 35 | +4 | +1.00 | 600 |
| Monica | Obstetric nursing | 38 | 35 | +3 | +0.75 | 575 |
| Thomas | Nursing of children | 36 | 35 | +1 | +0.25 | 525 |
| Paula | Psychiatric nursing | 33 | 35 | −2 | −0.50 | 450 |
| Erica | Medical nursing | 31 | 35 | −4 | −1.00 | 400 |
| Joanna | Nursing of children | 28 | 35 | −7 | −1.75 | 325 |

| Sequence of steps | Example |
|---|---|
| 1. Calculate the $z$-score. | In Table 5-15, the $z$-score is given for each raw score value. |
| 2. Multiply the $z$-score by 100. | For Arlene, the calculation is $+1.25 \times 100 = 125$. |
| 3. Add 500. | Thus, $125 + 500 = 625$. |

**Interpreting the Nursing Board Examination score.** To facilitate the interpretation of NBE scores calculated for Table 5-15, the following discussion of subtest results is presented.

| | Subtest | NBE | Discussion |
|---|---|---|---|
| Arlene | Medical nursing | 625 | This medical nursing score is above average — more than 1 standard deviation above the mean. |
| Irene | Surgical nursing | 600 | This surgical nursing score is also above average — exactly 1 standard deviation above the mean. |
| Monica | Obstetric nursing | 575 | This obstetric nursing score is also above average — 1¾ standard deviations above the mean. |
| Paula | Psychiatric nursing | 450 | This psychiatric nursing score is ½ standard deviation below the mean — still very acceptable, however. |
| Joanna | Nursing of children | 325 | This nursing-of-children score is failing or unacceptable; it is 1¾ standard deviations below the mean. An NBE score of 350 is a typical cutoff point for pass/fail. |

## Standard error of measurement

The standard error of measurement indicates how much Kristen's score would vary if she were tested repeatedly with the same test and no learning had occurred between tests. Error in measurement is always present in testing, so Kristen's score would not always be exactly the same. Although error in measurement cannot be eliminated, it can be estimated. By calculating the standard error of measurement, the nursing instructor can get a better indication of Kristen's true score.

The standard error of measurement can be calculated by using the standard deviation and the reliability of the test. The following formula is used:

$$SE_{meas} = s_x \sqrt{1 - r_{xx}}$$

where SE$_{meas}$ is the standard error of measurement, $s_x$ is the standard deviation of test X, and $r_{xx}$ is the reliability coefficient for test X.

If we apply this formula to a pharmacology examination that has a standard deviation of 6.14 and a reliability coefficient of 0.82, the following calculation results:

$$SE_{meas} = 6.14 \sqrt{1 - 0.82}$$
$$SE_{meas} = 6.14 \sqrt{0.18} = 6.14 \times 0.42 = 2.60$$

If Kristen receives a score of 69 on the final examination in pharmacology, and if the standard error of measurement for the examination is 2.60, Kristen's true score lies somewhere between 66.4 and 71.6 (69±2.60). If the standard error of measurement is considered by the instructor, the final grades for many borderline students such as Kristen may change. Many computer-scoring services cite the standard error of measurement on their item analysis printouts.

If the test has a large standard error of measurement, such as 9.6, Kristen's true score will be somewhere between 59.4 and 78.6. Obviously, this error range is so great that the instructor should throw out the test scores. In order to ultimately reduce the size of the standard error of measurement, the instructor would rewrite the test to improve its reliability and to decrease the standard deviation.

## Percentiles and percentile rank

Schools often report class rank for each member of the graduating class. Janet's class rank may be five (with only four students ahead of her). Her ranking, however, does not tell whether Janet ranks fifth out of 25 or fifth out of 250. This problem always occurs with rank. The discrepancy can be eliminated by using a percentage scale, so that the ranks reported have a similar meaning regardless of class size.

This section presents the conversion of metric or raw scores into a relative position score expressed as a percentage—the percentile rank.

- *Percentile rank* is that point in a distribution at or below which a given percentage of scores occurs.
- *Percentile* is a point on the measurement scale that divides the distribution into hundredths.

By definition, *percentile rank* is a percentage. It can never be negative or greater than 100. A percentile rank corresponds to an area of the frequency distribution, whereas a percentile is a score or a point in the base line of a frequency distribution. This is illustrated in Fig. 5-13.

It is important to be aware that when metric data (the raw test

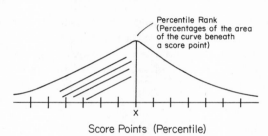

**Fig. 5-13.** Percentile rank and percentile.

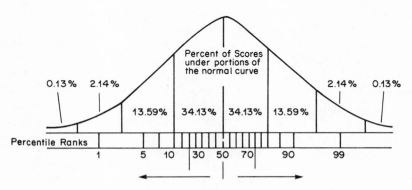

**Fig. 5-14.** Relationship of percentile rank to the normal curve.

scores) are converted into percentile ranks, the raw test score data are lost.

Percentile ranks are based only on the ranking of test scores. As a result, in a normal distribution percentile ranks tend to exaggerate the differences among the students at the extreme ends of the distribution. This is shown graphically in Fig. 5-14. In other words, the following statements are true for percentile rank in a normal distribution:

- The score distance corresponding to a given percentage (or area) increases as the distance from the center of the distribution increases.
- Similarly, the score distance corresponding to a given percentage (or area) decreases near the center of the distribution.

Table 5-16 illustrates the difference in score versus percentile distances as related to a normal distribution. These score and percentile differences have important implications for nursing educators who are

**Table 5-16.** Comparison of percentile rank and score differences

| Test results | Janet | Linda | Difference |
|---|---|---|---|
| Medical test | | | |
|   Percentile rank | 60 | 50 | 10 |
|   Test score | 64 | 60 | 4 |
| Surgical test | | | |
|   Percentile rank | 90 | 80 | 10 |
|   Test score | 79 | 72 | 7 |
| Psychiatric test | | | |
|   Percentile rank | 99 | 89 | 10 |
|   Test score | 95 | 78 | 17 |

interpreting percentile rank. For example, whereas the percentile rank differences between Janet's and Linda's medical test scores is ten, their actual score difference is only four. In contrast, whereas the percentile rank difference on Janet's and Linda's psychiatric test scores remains at ten, their actual test score difference is 17. Thus, their percentile rank difference remains constant, although their raw score test difference has become about four times as great. Given these limitations, we must be cautious about assuming that large differences in percentile rank correspond to large score differences.

Since information relative to percentile ranks is specific to the population, it is desirable to have norms on many different populations.

Suppose Sharon wants to transfer from an associate-degree nursing program to a baccalaureate-degree nursing program. If we tell Sharon she is at the eighty-fifth percentile rank of all entering transfer students into the four-year college, she may be pleased. However this population contains everyone transferring into the college (including many non-nursing majors). In contrast, if we tell Sharon her percentile rank derived from the population of transferring associate-degree nursing students is 75, she will have more relevant information and can be assured that her test score is above average for transferring nursing students.

**Directions for calculating percentile rank for a simple frequency distribution.** The percentile rank is computed in the following manner for ungrouped data:

$$P = \frac{cf + 0.5(fx)}{N} \times 100$$

**Table 5-17.** Percentile rank from ungrouped data

| Students | Score | cf | Percentile rank |
|----------|-------|-----|-----------------|
| Theresa | 88 | 10 | 95 |
| Janet | 84 | 9 | 85 |
| Betty | 80 | 8 | 75 |
| Mary | 79 | 7 | 65 |
| Paula | 77 | 6 | 55 |
| Michelle | 74 | 5 | 45 |
| Sharon | 68 | 4 | 35 |
| Nancy | 66 | 3 | 25 |
| Patricia | 65 | 2 | 15 |
| Stephanie | 61 | 1 | 5 |

where $P$ is the percentile rank, $cf$ is the cumulative frequency, $N$ is the number of scores in the distribution, and $fx$ is the frequency with which a particular raw score occurs. The following example indicates how to calculate the percentile rank(s) for the raw scores of 84 and 68 from Table 5-17.

| Sequence of steps | Examples | |
|-------------------|----------|--|
| 1. Determine how many students fall below the score in question. | In Table 5-17, $cf$ for score 84 is 8. | In Table 5-17, $cf$ for score 68 is 3. |
| 2. Determine the frequency with which the score in question occurs. | The score 84 occurs once. | The score 68 occurs once. |
| 3. Multiply 0.5 by the frequency determined in step 2. | $0.5 \times 1 = 0.5$ | $0.5 \times 1 = 0.5$ |
| 4. Add the cumulative frequency from step 1 to the information found in step 3. | $cf + 0.5(fx) =$ $8 + 0.5 = 8.5$ | $cf + 0.5(fx) =$ $3 + 0.5 = 3.5$ |
| 5. Divide the information in step 4 by the total number of students. | $\dfrac{8 + 0.5}{10} = 0.85$ | $\dfrac{3 + 0.5}{10} = 0.35$ |
| 6. Multiply by 100 to obtain the percentile rank. | $0.85 \times 100 = 85\%$ | $35 \times 100 = 35\%$ |

**Directions for calculating percentile rank for a grouped frequency distribution.** The percentile rank is computed in the following manner for grouped data:

**Table 5-18.** Grouped data from burn patient care examination scores

| Apparent score limits | Real score limits | Frequency | Cumulative frequency |
|---|---|---|---|
| 54-56 | 53.5-56.5 | 2 | 35 |
| 51-53 | 50.5-53.5 | 1 | 33 |
| 48-50 | 47.5-50.5 | 2 | 32 |
| 45-47 | 44.5-47.5 | 11 | 30 |
| 42-44 | 41.5-44.5 | 4 | 19 |
| 39-41 | 38.5-41.5 | 8 | 15 |
| 36-38 | 35.5-38.5 | 5 | 7 |
| 33-35 | 32.5-35.5 | 2 | 2 |

$$P = \frac{cf + \dfrac{x - LL}{i}\ (f)}{N} \times 100$$

where $P$ is the percentile rank, $cf$ is the cumulative frequency, $x$ is the raw score, $LL$ is the real lower limit of the interval, $i$ is the interval width, $f$ is the frequency of the interval, and $N$ is the total number of raw scores. The following example indicates how to calculate the percentile rank for the raw score of 46 from Table 5-18.

| Sequence of steps | Example |
|---|---|
| 1. Subtract the real lower limit of the interval from the raw score in question and divide the result by the interval width. | In Table 5-18: $\dfrac{46 - 44.5}{3.0} = \dfrac{1.5}{3.0} = 0.5$ |
| 2. Multiply the frequency of the interval by the number obtained in step 1. | $11 \times 0.5 = 5.5$ |
| 3. Add the cumulative frequency for those scores in the interval *below* the one in which the score in question occurs to the number obtained in step 2. | $19 + 5.5 = 24.5$ |
| 4. Divide the number obtained in step 3 by the number of scores in the distribution. | $\dfrac{24.5}{35} = 0.70$ |
| 5. Multiply the number obtained in step 4 by 100. | $0.70 \times 100 = 70$ |

**Disadvantages of percentile ranks.** Percentile ranks have a few disadvantages. They indicate only the rank of the student in the group without indicating the relationship of the student's raw score to the mean or to the standard deviation. Since percentile ranks are ranked data, not metric data, they are not subject to further mathematical manipulation: they cannot be added, subtracted, or averaged. For percentile ranks in a normal distribution, differences are exaggerated near the mean and minimized at the extreme ends of the distribution.

**Advantage of percentile ranks.** The primary advantage of percentile ranks is their ease of interpretation. For example, a percentile rank of 60 indicates that a student ranks *with or above* 60% of the students who took the test.

Some test publishers use percentile ranks of 0 to 100; others use 1 to 99. Theirs is a philosophical difference. The rationale for using 1 to 99 is that no individual can score *below* himself or herself and, similarly, no individual can score above himself or herself.

**The percentile band.** Percentile bands are commonly used by professional testing services to report test results. As the name suggests, the percentile band is a range of percentile ranks. The upper limit of the band is one standard error *above* the raw score, and the lower limit of the band is one standard error *below* the raw score. The primary purpose of reporting percentile bands is to emphasize the measurement error present in each score. It helps to remind everyone that test scores should not be treated as precise values.

### Describing relationships: correlation

One of the most common statistical measurements is the measurement of relationship between sets of data. Nursing educators and practitioners are often concerned with such relationships. For example, a nursing educator may be concerned with the relationship between a student's high school average and academic success in the nursing program. A pediatric nurse may be concerned with the relationship between a patient's weight and a drug dosage.

Correlation is concerned with measuring the relationship between two or more variables. Regression is concerned with measuring the degree of change in one variable (the dependent variable) associated with the change in one or more other variables (the independent variable). When the dependent variable increases as the independent variable increases, a *positive* relationship exists. When the dependent variable decreases as the independent variable increases, a *negative* relationship exists. A benefit of computing correlation is the ability to predict one variable if the value of the second variable is given.

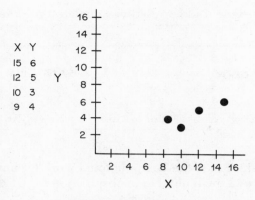

**Fig. 5-15.** Scattergram.

## *Scattergrams*

Scattergrams illustrate graphically the relationship between two sets of data. Fig. 5-15 illustrates a set of paired observations accompanied by a scattergram for the set of data.

### *Coefficient of correlation*

Correlation coefficients are briefly described in Chapter 4. The following assumes an understanding of that discussion.

Although the scattergram in Fig. 5-15 approximates the strength and direction of the relationship, it does not provide a precise correlation coefficient. By referring to Fig. 5-15, we can state that the relationship between $x$ and $y$ is positive and moderately strong. However, by using a computational formula, we can determine the exact correlation coefficient.

Computers are responsible for the frequent application of correlation measurements, especially multiple correlations.

**Directions for computing the coefficient of correlation.** The Pearson product-moment formula is a common method for computing correlation. The formula is:

$$r = \frac{n\,\Sigma xy - (\Sigma x)(\Sigma y)}{\sqrt{[n\,\Sigma x^2 - (\Sigma x)^2][n\,\Sigma y^2 - (\Sigma y)^2]}}$$

where $r$ is the product-moment correlation coefficient, $n$ is the number of pairs of scores, $x$ represents each of the raw scores on the first variable, and $y$ represents each of the raw scores on the second variable. Table 5-19 illustrates the correlation coefficients depicted graphi-

**Table 5-19.** Coefficient of correlation calculated from raw scores

| $x$ | $y$ | $xy$ | $x^2$ | $y^2$ |
|---|---|---|---|---|
| 15 | 6 | 90 | 225 | 36 |
| 12 | 5 | 60 | 144 | 25 |
| 10 | 3 | 30 | 100 | 9 |
| 9 | 4 | 36 | 81 | 16 |
| $\Sigma x = 46$ | $\Sigma y = 18$ | $\Sigma xy = 216$ | $\Sigma x^2 = 550$ | $\Sigma y^2 = 86$ |

cally in Fig. 5-15. Since the computational work is cumbersome, the example involves a small number of observations.

| Sequence of steps | Example |
|---|---|
| 1. Multiply the number of pairs of scores by the sum of all multiplied pairs. | In Table 5-19, $4 \times 216 = 864$. |
| 2. Multiply the sum of all raw scores on the first variable by the sum of all scores on the second variable, and subtract the product from the product calculated in step 1. | $46 \times 18 = 828$ <br> $864 - 828 = 36$ |
| 3. Multiply the number of pairs of scores by the sum of all squared scores on the first variable; then subtract the squared sum of all scores on the first variable. | $4 \times 550 = 2,200$ <br> $2,200 - 2,116 = 84$ |
| 4. Multiply the number of pairs of scores by the sum of all squared scores on the second variable; then subtract the squared sum of all scores on the second variable. | $4 \times 86 = 344$ <br> $344 - 324 = 20$ |
| 5. Take the square root of the product of the result in steps 3 and 4. | $\sqrt{84 \times 20} = \sqrt{1,680} = 40.9$ |
| 6. Divide the result of step 2 by the result of step 5. | $36 \div 40.9 = +0.87$ |

The exact correlation coefficient is +0.87. Now not only do we know that there is a high degree of relationship between $x$ and $y$; we also know the exact correlation coefficient existing between $x$ and $y$.

The Pearson product-moment correlation is relatively simple to

**Table 5-20.** Coefficient of correlation calculated from $z$-scores

| $z_x$ | $z_y$ | $z_x z_y$ |
|---|---|---|
| +1.59 | −0.02 | −0.03 |
| +0.95 | −0.01 | −0.01 |
| −0.05 | +1.01 | −0.05 |
| −1.67 | +2.00 | −3.34 |
| | | $\Sigma$ −3.43 |

compute for a distribution of $z$-scores. The following formula is used:

$$r = \frac{\Sigma z_x z_y}{N}$$

where $r$ is the Pearson product-moment correlation, $z_x$ is a $z$-score plotted on the $x$-axis, $z_y$ is a $z$-score plotted on the $y$-axis, and $N$ is the number of raw scores.

| Sequence of steps | Example |
|---|---|
| 1. Multiply each $z$-score on the $x$-axis by its score on the $y$-axis; then add all the products. | In Table 5-20, −0.03 + −0.01 + −0.05 + −3.34 = −3.43. |
| 2. Divide the result of step 1 by the number of raw scores. | −3.43 ÷ 4 = −0.85 |

### Interpreting correlation

It is difficult to state with certainty that any specific correlation coefficient is strong, moderately strong, weak, or relatively weak. Such a determination depends on what is being compared. For example, a correlation of + 0.40 is weak for two reading test scores. However, if we are comparing two characteristics that apparently have nothing in common, such as sudden infant death and geographic location, a correlation of + 0.40 may be very significant and worth further study.

There are also statistical considerations one should keep in mind when attempting to draw inferences from correlations. For example, correlation is directly related to the variability (standard deviation) of each set of scores. Therefore, two variables are unlikely to move in correlation with each other if the standard deviation of one (or both) is large.

When we interpret a correlation between two variables, it is not correct to infer that one variable causes the other. Although this possibility exists, many other variables may also be factors. For example,

**Table 5-21.** Matrix of intercorrelations

| Tests | Tests | | | |
| | A | B | C | D |
| --- | --- | --- | --- | --- |
| B | 0.22 | | | |
| C | 0.31 | 0.42 | | |
| D | 0.43 | 0.33 | 0.46 | |
| E | 0.60 | 0.66 | 0.78 | 0.75 |

certain native peoples believed that wearing garlic around their necks protected them from malaria. In reality, the garlic protected them from mosquito bites, thus protecting them from malaria. Thus, it was inferred that X caused Y based on the relationship of X and Y; in reality, X was affected by Z.

In contrast, to say that we cannot attribute causality on the basis of correlation is not the same as to say we cannot make predictions based on correlations. For example, it is possible to use the concept of correlation to predict that natives who wear garlic will not get malaria. However, the correlation concept cannot be used to make statements about causality.

In summary, correlation coefficients are very useful in providing information about students and testing protocols. However, they should be cautiously interpreted by the teacher.

### *Multiple correlations*

Simple correlation involves measuring the correlation between two variables. Multiple correlation involves measuring the relationship or relationships between two or more variables (more than one independent variable).

Multivariate analysis (the correlation of many variables) has become common with the use of computer technology. This technology has made mathematical calculations efficient, accurate, and relatively easy. Following is a brief discussion of multiple correlation.

Table 5-21 illustrates the multiple correlation among five tests. There is a very low correlation between tests A and B (0.22). There is also a low correlation between tests A and C (0.31) and tests B and C (0.42). Similarly, a low correlation exists between tests A and D, B and D, and C and D. In sharp contrast, there is a strong relationship between tests A and E (0.60), B and E (0.66), C and E (0.78), and D and E (0.75).

Table 5-22 represents a hypothetical matrix of correlations be-

**Table 5-22.** Hypothetical matrix of intercorrelations between the NBE subtests

|  | Medical | Surgical | Obstetric | Nursing of children | Psychiatric |
|---|---|---|---|---|---|
| **Medical** | 1.00 | | | | |
| **Surgical** | 0.78 | | | | |
| **Obstetric** | 0.68 | 0.55 | | | |
| **Nursing of children** | 0.53 | 0.59 | 0.80 | | |
| **Psychiatric** | 0.19 | 0.33 | 0.31 | 0.28 | 1.00 |

tween the five subtests on the NBE. What conclusions might we draw from the data?

The subtest scores on the NBE differ in their degree of correlation. For example:

- There is a relatively high intercorrelation between the medical and surgical nursing subtests (+ 0.78).
- There is a high intercorrelation between the nursing-of-children and obstetric nursing subtests (+ 0.80).
- In contrast, there are very low intercorrelations between the psychiatric nursing subtest and the medical, surgical, obstetric, and nursing-of-children subtests. The intercorrelations are as follows: psychiatric nursing and medical nursing (+ 0.19), psychiatric nursing and surgical nursing (+ 0.33), psychiatric nursing and obstetric nursing (+ 0.31), psychiatric nursing and nursing of children (+ 0.28).

## The $t$-test statistic

The $t$-test statistic is briefly discussed in this chapter since it appears in the computer analysis printout in Chapter 6. Although most teachers ignore this measure, an understanding of the statistic may be helpful.

To use the $t$ statistic effectively, we must assume that: (1) the test scores are normally distributed and (2) the samples have equal variances.

### The t-test

The $t$-test is a test of significance between two sample means. Two different formulas are used for computing the $t$-test, and two rationales apply to it:

1. Test for independent means. This $t$-test is used to compare two

means that are unrelated (when the means have been calculated on two samples drawn from two different populations). (For example, sample 1 may consist of NBE scores from school A and sample 2 of NBE scores from school B.)
2. Test for dependent means. This *t*-test is used to compare two means that are matched or related (when two means are obtained for a single group). For example, we may wish to test the hypothesis that there is no significant difference between the pretest and posttest scores on a particular teacher-made test.

To keep this discussion informative but nonmathematical, the formulas are not illustrated or discussed, but interpretation of the resulting *t*, as it appears in research articles, is presented.

To determine if a significant difference exists between the two means, the *t* table is used. For effective use of this table, two values must be obtained: the level of significance and the degree of freedom *(df)*.

The degree of freedom is the number of independent observations for a source of variation minus the number of independent parameters estimated in computing the variation. The number of independent observations merely means the number of subjects in the study. For example, if there are 30 subjects, the number of independent observations is 30. A parameter is merely a measure computed from all observations in a population. For example, a population mean is a parameter.

**Test for independent means.** Suppose a dean wishes to determine if there is any significant difference between the NBE scores for surgical nursing at one school (school A) and the NBE scores for surgical nursing at another school (school B).

Such a check does not involve individual matching or related means. The two groups are separate and, consequently, independent groups. Furthermore, each class contains 15 students, and the obtained *t* is 3.30 (at a 0.01 level of significance). To determine the degree of freedom for a *t*-test for independent means, the number of cases minus one in the first sample is added to the number of cases minus one in the second sample: $(N_1 - 1) + (N_2 - 1)$, or $(N_1 + N_2 - 2)$. The degree of freedom for these independent samples of students each is: $(N_1 + N_2 - 2) = (15 + 15 - 2) = 28$. By referring to Table 5-23, we see that the *t* value when $df = 28$ (with a 0.01 level of significance) is 2.763. This obtained *t* value would occur only 1% of the time by chance. Since the obtained *t* was 3.30, greater than 2.763, a significant difference exists between the surgical nursing scores at school A and those at school B.

**Table 5-23.** Values of $t$ at the 0.05 and 0.01 levels of significance

| Degree of freedom *(df)* | Value of $t$ | |
|:---:|:---:|:---:|
| | **0.05 Level of significance** | **0.01 Level of significance** |
| 1 | 12.706 | 63.657 |
| 2 | 4.303 | 9.925 |
| 3 | 3.182 | 5.841 |
| 4 | 2.776 | 4.604 |
| 5 | 2.571 | 4.032 |
| 6 | 2.447 | 3.707 |
| 7 | 2.365 | 3.499 |
| 8 | 2.306 | 3.355 |
| 9 | 2.262 | 3.250 |
| 10 | 2.228 | 3.169 |
| 11 | 2.201 | 3.106 |
| 12 | 2.179 | 3.055 |
| 13 | 2.160 | 3.012 |
| 14 | 2.145 | 2.977 |
| 15 | 2.131 | 2.947 |
| 16 | 2.120 | 2.921 |
| 17 | 2.110 | 2.898 |
| 18 | 2.101 | 2.878 |
| 19 | 2.093 | 2.861 |
| 20 | 2.086 | 2.845 |
| 21 | 2.080 | 2.831 |
| 22 | 2.074 | 2.819 |
| 23 | 2.069 | 2.807 |
| 24 | 2.064 | 2.797 |
| 25 | 2.060 | 2.787 |
| 26 | 2.056 | 2.779 |
| 27 | 2.052 | 2.771 |
| 28 | 2.048 | 2.763 |
| 29 | 2.045 | 2.756 |
| 30 | 2.042 | 2.750 |

**Test for dependent means.** The degree of freedom for a $t$ statistic calculated for dependent means is equal to $n - 1$, where $n$ is the number of pairs of scores. Suppose the obtained $t$ for 30 students on the pretest and posttest in pharmacology is reported as 4.3 (at a 0.05 level of significance). In Table 5-23, the $t$ value when $df$ is 29 ($n - 1$, or $30 - 1$), at a 0.05 level of significance, is 2.045. Since the $t$ obtained was 4.3, greater than 2.045, a significant difference exists between the two means, and the obtained $t$ value would occur only 5% of the time by chance. Therefore, there was a significant difference between the pre-test and posttest scores in pharmacology.

In summary, the *t* statistic is merely a test used to determine if a significant difference exists between two means.

**Interpretation of the *t*-test.** A small group of nursing instructors are convinced that a basic knowledge of medical terminology is necessary for students to be able to read and interpret patients' progress reports; however, students usually have insufficient lecture time for this topic. The faculty decide to conduct "action research," a term applied to research done within a specific department to provide data for curriculum revision. The faculty decide to lecture on medical terminology to group A and to use a programmed text for group B and then test each group. The results follow:

|  | Mean | Standard deviation |
|---|---|---|
| Class A (following lecture) | 23.6 | 8.4 |
| Class B (following use of programmed text) | 26.4 | 8.4 |

$$N = 30$$
$$df = 28$$
$$\text{Obtained } t = 3.07$$

Class A has a final test mean of 23.6, and class B has a final test mean of 26.4. The nursing faculty must now ask themselves: Is the difference between the two classes important? Statistically speaking, is there a significant difference between the means? Remember that the *t*-test for independent means answers this question; note that the obtained *t* is 3.07. Table 5-23 shows that, at the 0.05 level of significance and 28 degrees of freedom, the table value of *t* is 2.048. Since the obtained *t* was 3.07, greater than 2.048, the faculty can conclude that teaching medical terminology with a programmed text is an acceptable educational alternative.

## SUMMARY

Raw scores from either teacher-made or standardized tests are merely a mass of unorganized data. These scores must be ordered for ease of inspection and presentation. Simple and grouped frequency distributions, as well as histograms and polygons, are frequently constructed to serve as summaries and graphic representations of test scores. Whereas frequency distributions and graphs are useful for providing an overall view of the distribution of test scores, measures of central tendency (that is, mean, mode, and median) are useful in describing the midpoint of the score distribution. The selection and use of any measure of central tendency are dependent on the nature of the data. To further describe test scores, measures of dispersion (or variability) describe the extent to which test scores are scattered or are clustered together. The most common measures of variability are range, variance, and standard deviation. The standard deviation is often the preferred measure of variability.

Standard scores, such as $z$-scores, $T$-scores, and NBE scores, are derived scores with known arithmetic means and standard deviations. They allow the comparison of the performance of an individual with the performance of other individuals on the same test. They also allow for comparison of students among test distributions. In contrast to standard scores, percentile ranks only indicate the rank of a student in the group without indicating the relationship of the student's raw score to the mean or to the standard deviation. Percentile ranks are not subject to further mathematical manipulation.

Correlation helps describe the relationship that exists between two variables. However, when interpreting a correlation, it is not correct to infer that one variable causes the other. Although this possibility exists, many other variables may also be factors. Correlation does not mean causation.

The $t$-test is a statistic used to determine if an important difference exists between two sample means. A $t$-test for independent means is used to compare two means that are unrelated. A $t$-test for dependent means is used to compare two means that are matched or related.

Interpreting test scores is a responsibility of every nursing instructor. Consequently, an understanding of the meaning of test scores is essential as we plan, implement, and evaluate instruction.

**REFERENCES**

Armitage, P.: Statistical methods in medical research, New York, 1971, John Wiley & Sons, Inc.
Avenso, F. J., and Cheifetz, P. M.: Elementary statistics through problem solving, Baltimore, 1974, The Williams & Wilkins Co.
Games, P. A., and Klare, D. R.: Elementary statistics, New York, 1967, McGraw-Hill Book Co., Inc.
Gellman, E. S.: Descriptive statistics for teachers, New York, 1973, Harper and Row Publishers, Inc.
Green, J. A.: Teacher-made tests, ed. 2, New York, 1975, Harper and Row.
Koosis, D. J.: Statistics, New York, 1971, John Wiley & Sons, Inc.
Lindquist, E. F., editor: Educational measurement, ed. 5, Washington, D.C., 1963, American Council on Education.
Lyman, H. B.: Test scores and what they mean, Englewood Cliffs, N.J., 1963, Prentice-Hall, Inc.

Minium, E. W.: Statistical reasoning in psychology and education, New York, 1970, John Wiley & Sons, Inc.

Townsend, E. A., and Burke, P. J.: Using statistics in classroom instruction, New York, 1975, The Macmillan Co.

Tyler, L. E.: Tests and measurements, Englewood Cliffs, N. J., 1963, Prentice-Hall, Inc.

Wallen, N. E.: Educational research; a guide to the process, Belmont, Calif.; 1974, Wadsworth.

# 6

# Item analysis

Standards and quality controls exist for the development of measurement instruments. By monitoring their instruments, test developers can make improvements when needed. This chapter focuses on the evaluation of instructor-made tests after they have been written, administered, and scored.

Evaluation of an assessment instrument can focus on individual test items or on the test as a whole. It can focus on such concepts as validity and reliability. The primary purpose of this discussion is to present a formalized procedure for assessing *individual* test items. This procedure — item analysis — ultimately contributes to the validity and reliability of an entire test.

## PURPOSES OF ITEM ANALYSIS
### Improve the assessment instrument

The primary purpose for evaluating any instrument is to improve it. Item analysis procedures can help identify item difficulty, item discriminating power, and the effectiveness of each distracter. When item analysis is completed, the test developer can take direct action to revise the test items that need improvement. Each revision contributes to the overall improvement of the test.

### Facilitate learning

Item analysis provides valuable information for future classroom activities. The teacher can learn to take more time explaining the concepts covered by the difficult items. The teacher can eliminate seriously defective items from the test, instead of defending them as fair. Thus, learning can be clarified, and individual test items can be rewritten and improved.

Item analysis information can provide indicators of students' strengths and weaknesses. This information can assist the instructor and the student in planning remedial activities. For example, during a review of response patterns to items in a pediatric nursing examination, it is determined that Marlene answered correctly all of the items related to nursing care for children with congenital heart disease. However, she missed almost every item on muscular dystrophy. Consequently, Marlene's teacher can use the item analysis data to individualize remedial instruction for Marlene.

### Improve teaching effectiveness

If a large percentage of the class incorrectly answered the items concerning muscular dystrophy, item analysis information could provide valuable cues to the instructor concerning the effectiveness of this unit's lessons. Perhaps the instructor spends too little time on the topic. The instructor possibly fails to provide concrete clinical examples. Based on the judgments of the instructor and recommendations from the students, the unit can be redeveloped. Thus, item analysis provides information for improving teaching effectiveness.

### Provide statistical information

When instructor-made tests are computer-scored, additional statistical information is provided. For example, internal consistency reliability, standard error of measurement, mean, median, and standard deviation are frequently calculated. In addition, percentile rank and $z$-scores are often provided. The interpretation of these statistical indices is discussed in Chapter 5. By reviewing these indices, the instructor receives information beyond specific item analysis data that will help improve the assessment instrument and will aid in grading.

### Increase instructor skill in test construction

As instructors apply the information provided by item analysis data (discrimination index, item difficulty, analysis of response patterns), their overall skill in test construction improves. This skill will contribute to the overall improvement in the assessment procedures for the entire nursing program.

## INTERPRETING ITEM ANALYSIS INDICES

Item analysis procedures focus on two basic statistical indices: a difficulty, or "easiness," index and a discriminating index.

### Difficulty index

The difficulty index is the percentage of students tested who answer the item correctly; that is:

$$P = \frac{N_r}{N_t}(100)$$

where $P$ is the percentage of students answering the item correctly
(difficulty index), $N_r$ is the number of students answering the item correctly, and $N_t$ is the total number of students who attempted to answer
the item.

### Example

An item on a classroom test is answered correctly by 21 of the 28 students who attempted to answer it. The level of difficulty is found as follows:

$$P = \frac{N_r}{N_t}(100) = \frac{21}{28}(100) = 75$$

Consequently, 75% of the students attempting the item answered it correctly.

Some measurement specialists suggest calling this index an easiness index because, as a difficulty index, it is numerically backward:
the higher the numerical value, the lower the difficulty. For example,
in the illustration just presented, 21 out of 28 students answered the
item correctly resulting in an item "difficulty" of 75%. In reality, the
item was easy. In contrast, the "easiness" index has a direct numerical
relationship rather than an inverted relationship and is easier to remember and use.

### Discrimination index

The discrimination index is a measure of how well an item discriminates between high achievers and low achievers on the test. It is
based on the assumption that the total test is logically a better indicator of performance than any of the individual items. In essence, the
discrimination index provides an indicator of how a specific test item
correlates with the total test score. This use of the total test score as
the criterion for classifying students into high scorers and low scorers,
followed by the use of these groups to calculate a discrimination index, is known as the internal consistency method of computing a discrimination index (Ahmann and Glock, 1971).

The rationale behind computation of an index of discrimination is
quite simple. A test item with maximum discriminating power would
result in every student in the upper group answering correctly and
every student in the lower group answering incorrectly. It is unrealistic to expect items to discriminate perfectly. In the typical test item,
some of the high scorers will answer correctly, and some of the low
scorers will answer correctly.

The following is a simplified formula for computing an item's discrimination power:

$$D = \frac{U - L}{N}$$

Where $D$ is the discrimination index, $U$ is the number of students in upper group answering *correctly*, $L$ is the number of students in lower group answering *correctly*, and $N$ is the number of students *in each* of the two groups.

**Example**

Suppose 10 of 12 students in the high group answered an item correctly. In contrast, 5 of 12 students in the low group answered the item correctly. The discriminating power for this test item would be:

$$D = \frac{10 - 5}{12} = +0.42$$

**Example**

Suppose 12 of 12 students in the high group answered an item correctly. In contrast, none of the 12 students in the low group answered the item correctly. The discrimination index would be:

$$D = \frac{12 - 0}{12} = +1.00$$

From this example, it is apparent that an index of $+1.00$ represents the maximum discriminating power.

**Example**

Suppose none of the 12 students in the high group answered correctly. In contrast, all 12 of the 12 students in the low group answered the item correctly. In this case, the discrimination index would be:

$$D = \frac{0 - 12}{12} = -1.00$$

From this example, it is apparent that $-1.00$ represents the minimum discriminating power.

It should now be obvious that the maximum value of the discrimination index is $+1.00$ and the minimum value is $-1.00$. Items with positive discrimination indices are desirable, since the high scorers are answering correctly. In contrast, items with negative discrimination indices are undesirable, since the low scorers are answering correctly, whereas the high scorers are missing the item.

Generally, the larger the positive value, the better the item. It is difficult to rigidly establish acceptable levels of discrimination, however. Even educational psychologists vary in their recommendations. For instructor-made tests, the following definitions may serve as a guide:

- If the discrimination index is 0.40 or greater, consider the item an "excellent" item.

- If the discrimination index is from 0.19 to .39, consider the item a "satisfactory" item.
- If the discrimination index is from 0.15 to 0.18, consider the item an "acceptable" item.
- A discrimination index below 0.15 indicates a "poor" item. (Throw out all items with negative values.)

To summarize, a *positively* discriminating item is:

- Answered correctly by those who scored high on the total test.
- Answered incorrectly by those who scored low on the total test.

A *negatively* discriminating item is:

- Answered correctly by those who scored low on the total test.
- Answered incorrectly by those who scored high on the total test.

## MANUAL ITEM ANALYSIS

If test-scoring services are available, they can provide a more accurate analysis than can be computed by hand, and in much less time. However, if these services are unavailable, the following procedure can be used to provide item analysis information for small classes (20 to 40 students):

1. Arrange all test papers from highest to lowest, based on the number of correct items per paper.
2. Divide the papers into the half with the highest scores and the half with the lowest scores, keeping all papers in descending order. (If you have an odd number of students, discard the middle paper.) For computer scoring, Brennan (1972) recommends that the high-score group contain 27% of the total and the low-score group contain 27%. However, if the class is extremely small, 50% of the students should be included in each group.
3. Using a sample work sheet like that shown in Table 6-1, put the total grade of each paper in the left-hand column, beginning at the top with the paper that has the highest grade. When the highest 50% has been listed, jump to the lower half of the table and list the lower 50%.
4. Take the highest paper and record an X under each item missed. The X's for each paper will run horizontally across the graph. Repeat this operation for each paper in the class.
5. When all the missed items are recorded, simply count vertically the number of X's tabulated under each item for the high 50% *and* for the low 50%. Space to record these data is provided above each item number.
6. If the number of misses in the high 50% equals or exceeds the misses in the low 50%, the item discriminates in favor of the lower-scoring students and we may assume that the question

**Table 6-1.** Work sheet for manual tabulation of item analysis

| | | | | | | | | | | |
|---|---|---|---|---|---|---|---|---|---|---|
| High 50% | 3 | 1 | 0 | 2 | 1 | 1 | 0 | 0 | 1 | 0 |
| Low 50% | 5 | 3 | 4 | 0 | 1 | 5 | 0 | 5 | 0 | 3 |
| Item →<br>Score ↴ | 1 | 2 | 3 | 4 | 5 | 6 | 7 | 8 | 9 | 10 |
| **Upper 50%** | | | | | | | | | | |
| 1 Kelly | X | | | | | | | | | |
| 2 Kristen | X | | | X | | | | | | |
| 3 Amy | X | | | X | | | | | | |
| 4 Janet | | X | | | X | | | | | |
| 5 Marie | | | | | | X | | | X | |
| **Lower 50%** | | | | | | | | | | |
| 1 Rebecca | X | | X | | | X | | X | | |
| 2 Diane | X | | X | | | X | | X | | X |
| 3 Stephanie | X | X | X | | | X | | X | | |
| 4 Joel | X | X | X | | | X | | X | | X |
| 5 David | X | X | | | X | X | | X | | X |

has some defect: for example, it may be ambiguous. Circle such items. Now look up the circled items on your test and either omit or revise them.

The discrimination index can be calculated for sample items from Table 6-1 in the following manner:

| Item | Item discrimination | Discussion |
|---|---|---|
| 1 | $D = \dfrac{2 - 0}{5} = +0.4$ | For item 1, two students from the top 50% of the class answered correctly, and none from the bottom 50% of the class answered correctly. Consequently, the item discriminated in favor of the high scorers. |
| 3 | $D = \dfrac{5 - 1}{5} = +0.8$ | For item 3, five students from the top 50% of the class answered correctly, and only one student from the bottom 50% of the class answered correctly. Consequently, the item strongly discriminated in favor of the high scorers. |

| Item | Item discrimination | Discussion |
|------|--------------------|------------|
| 4 | $D = \dfrac{3-5}{5} = -0.4$ | For item 4, three students from the top 50% of the class answered correctly, and five students from the bottom 50% of the class answered correctly. Consequently, the item has a negative discrimination index. It discriminates in favor of the low scorers. The instructor should eliminate or rewrite this item. |
| 5 | $D = \dfrac{4-4}{5} = 0.0$ | For item 5, four high scorers and four low scorers answered the item correctly. Consequently, the item has a zero discrimination index. |
| 8 | $D = \dfrac{5-0}{5} = +1.00$ | For item 5, all the high scorers answered correctly, and all the low scorers answered incorrectly. Consequently, the item perfectly discriminates between the high and low scorers. (In practice, this is fairly rare.) |

The difficulty index can also be calculated for sample items from Table 6-1 in the following manner:

| Item | Item difficulty index | Discussion |
|------|----------------------|------------|
| 1 | $P = \dfrac{2}{10} = 20\%$ | For item 1, two students out of ten answered correctly. Consequently, the item is a hard item, with a corresponding low difficulty index. |
| 4 | $P = \dfrac{8}{10} = 80\%$ | For item 4, eight students out of ten answered correctly. Consequently, the item is an easy item, with a corresponding high difficulty index. |
| 7 | $P = \dfrac{10}{10} = 100\%$ | For item 7, all the students answered correctly. Consequently, the item is a very easy item, with the maximum difficulty index. |
| 8 | $P = \dfrac{5}{10} = 50\%$ | For item 8, five students answered correctly. Consequently, the item is of medium difficulty. |

## COMPUTER OUTPUT FOR ITEM ANALYSIS

Computer output for item analysis of one sample test item is illustrated in the following example. The format may vary, but the same variables should be present.

**Example**

Mrs. Smith, 55 years old, is admitted to the hospital with a diagnosis of advanced arteriosclerosis and congestive heart failure. She is edematous, cyanotic, short of breath, restless, and nervous. Her pulse is rapid, weak, and irregular. Her blood pressure is 180/110. The following orders are written by the physician:

> Phenobarbital 30 mg tid
> Digoxin 0.25 mg STAT and then 0.125 mg daily PO
> Lasix 40 mg bid
> KCl 10% Sol 10cc tid

Which drug would you administer first?

1. Digoxin
2. KCl
3. Lasix
4. Phenobarbital

### Item Analysis Data

Below is the computer output illustrating the item analysis data for the test item shown in this example.

| Item | 11 | Keyed resp. | 4 |
|---|---|---|---|
| Difficulty | 35 | Discr. | 0.47 |
| Pt. BISRL | 0.66 | T | 3.37 |
| *Mean score rights* | 25.3 | *Mean score wrongs* | 21.1 |

Response patterns (for upper and lower halves of score distribution)

| Response | 1 | 2 | 3 | 4 | Omits | 1 | 2 | 3 | 4 | Omits |
|---|---|---|---|---|---|---|---|---|---|---|
| By high scorers | 3 | 0 | 0 | 5 | 0 | 17.6 | 0.0 | 0.0 | 29.4 | 0.0 |
| By low scorers | 5 | 0 | 3 | 1 | 0 | 29.4 | 0.0 | 17.6 | 5.9 | 0.0 |
| | | | **Number** | | | | | **Percent** | | |

### Description

| Item | 11 | The particular test item under consideration (i.e., test item example 1). |
|---|---|---|
| Keyed Resp | 4 | The correct answer for item 11. |
| Difficulty | 35 | Percentage of students answering the question correctly. |
| Discr | 0.47 | A measure of item discrimination. |
| Pt. BISRL | 0.66 | A sophisticated index of discriminating power often used by professional test developers;° a correlation between item score and total test score. |

°For a more detailed explanation, see Lindquist, E. F., editor: Educational measurement, Washington, D.C., 1951, American Council on Education, reprint ed. 5, Menasha, Wis., 1963, George Banta.

**Description**

| | | |
|---|---|---|
| T | 3.37 | A statistic to determine if the point biserial correlation differs significantly from zero. An item test statistic indicating a measure of an item's discriminating power, it is computed by calculating the difference between the percentages of the upper and lower groups that answered the item correctly. |
| *Mean score rights* | 25.3 | The average, or mean, score for the six students, or the 35.3% of the class, that answered the item correctly. (Note: This mean score is derived by averaging the scores of the 29.4% of the high scorers and the 5.9% of the low scorers.) |
| *Mean score wrongs* | 21.1 | The average, or mean, score for the 11 students, of 64.6% of the class, that answered the item incorrectly. (Note: This mean score is derived by averaging the scores for the 17.6% of the high scorers and the 47.0% [29.4 + 17.6] of the low scorers.) |

Observe that the index of difficulty (35%) and the discriminating power of the test item (+0.47) are very acceptable. This item is a very difficult item, since only 29.4% of the high scorers and only 5.9% of the low scorers answered correctly. The difficulty index, the percentage of students answering the question correctly, is approximately 35% (29.4% + 5.9%). The response patterns explain more than the difficulty index. They show the percentage of high scorers answering correctly, the percentage of low scorers answering correctly, and the percentages of students responding to each distracter.

The item discriminates well (D = +0.47). Five high scorers answered correctly, and only one low scorer answered correctly. In addition, two of the three distracters were effective. Eight students chose distracter 1, and three students chose distracter 3. Furthermore, the first distracter has a differential attractiveness: that is, it is more attractive to the lower scorers than to the higher scorers. Notice that three high scorers chose this option whereas five low scorers chose it. In this way, the first distracter contributes to the discrimination power of the test item. The third distracter also has a high differential attractiveness, since only low scorers chose this distracter.

## TEST ITEM FILE

The instructor may wish to use a test item file as a permanent record of items for possible use in later examinations. Information obtained from the item analysis can be recorded on an item card like that shown in Fig. 6-1. The card may be any convenient size. Even blank or used keypunch cards make good test item cards. The item card con-

```
┌─────────────────────────────────────────────────────────────────────────┐
│ Item                                                                      │
│                                                                           │
│                                                                           │
│                                                                           │
│                                                                           │
│                                                                           │
│ Course        _____                                                 │
│                                                                           │
│ Unit          _____                                                 │
│                                                                           │
│ Obj. #        _____              Difficulty        _____      │
│                                                                           │
│ Taxonomy    _____                Discrimination  _____        │
└─────────────────────────────────────────────────────────────────────────┘
```

**Fig. 6-1.** Sample item file card.

tains not only a copy of the individual test item: more important, it provides descriptive information about the item.

Item cards can be filed according to units of instruction. For example, a course on medical-surgical nursing may be divided into the following units:

Unit 1 — Diseases of the Respiratory System
Unit 2 — Diseases of the Gastrointestinal System
Unit 3 — Diseases of the Musculoskeletal System
Unit 4 — Diseases of the Nervous System
•Unit 5 — Diseases of the Endocrine System

All test items for Unit 1 would be filed together. The instructor might wish to further sort the cards according to taxonomy: for Unit 1, for example, all the questions measuring the knowledge domain could be filed together, all the items measuring comprehension could be filed together, and so on.

When test item files are used with a table of specifications, the mechanics of preparing a test for typing are relatively simple. This combination also ensures high test content validity and simplifies the preparation of parallel forms of the test.

The primary limitation of a test item file is the initial time involved in recording the necessary information. However, as the instructor continues to write test items and develops a fairly large number of test items for each unit of instruction, the time required for actual test construction decreases.

## LIMITATIONS OF ITEM ANALYSIS
## FOR TEACHER-MADE TESTS
### Distortion from limited class size

Item analysis procedures for instructor-made tests are usually based on a limited number of students. Consequently, a shift of one response from one option to another will change the discrimination and difficulty indices. Unlike item analysis data for standardized achievement tests, based on hundreds of cases, item analysis data based on small numbers should be considered an estimation. Classroom test makers, therefore, should use careful professional judgment when making decisions regarding item retention or revision.

### Potential conflict with content validity

If a low or negative discrimination index results in deletion of an item, the content validity of the test could be reduced. Items should be redeveloped with this in mind. If the table of specifications is seriously considered when decisions regarding item deletion are made, the content validity will remain high. When forced to choose between keeping a test item with a relatively low discrimination index and the reduction of content validity, the instructor should give content validity higher priority.

### Inapplicability to essay tests

It is extremely difficult to apply item analysis techniques to essay items. Reliable scoring of essay items is difficult to achieve; even the attempt to achieve it is extremely time-consuming. Obviously, restricted responses scored by the analytical method are the most practical for item analysis.

In practice, essay items rarely are carefully analyzed for teacher-made tests. The time involved and the questions concerning reliability make the practice too inefficient.

## ITEM ANALYSIS FOR CRITERION-REFERENCED TESTS

To understand the role of item analysis in criterion-referenced testing, we must understand the role of mastery tests and formative and summative evaluation. A mastery test is a criterion-referenced measurement used in formative and summative evaluation.

*Formative evaluation* is a term first used by Scriven (1967) to refer to brief diagnostic progress tests used to determine whether a student has mastered a unit of instruction. Frequent formative evaluation tests pace the student's learning and help keep the student motivated. If the instructor is presenting material based on a hierarchical classification of knowledge (simple to more complex learning), formative tests also help ensure that lower-level learning is mastered before higher-level learning is attempted. Some educators believe formative tests should be ungraded and only marked for mastery or nonmastery.

In contrast to formative evaluation, summative evaluation consists of a test at the end of a term for purposes such as (1) grading student performance, (2) certifying students, and (3) evaluating curriculum effectiveness. The Nursing Board Examination is, for example, a summative evaluation.

Criterion-referenced tests are appropriate for formative and summative evaluation because they allow for a dichotomous, yes or no decision regarding the student's mastery status.

Popham and Husek (1969) criticize the use of norm-referenced measurement techniques for the analysis of criterion-referenced examinations. Their major criticism is based on the dependence of norm-referenced measurement on score variability. They argue that, since after sufficient instruction a good criterion-referenced test should result in little score variability, new, criterion-referenced concepts relative to item analysis are needed. For example, in norm-referenced item analysis, an item with a low discrimination index is considered inadequate. In contrast, in a criterion-referenced examination, an item answered correctly by everyone is seen as ideal.

The concepts of item discrimination and item difficulty must also be viewed differently for criterion-referenced measures. Although item analysis techniques for criterion-referenced instruction are still in an early stage of their development, a professional dialogue, with accompanying research, has begun on this topic.

Two approaches to item analysis for criterion-referenced instruction are briefly reviewed below. Other approaches are being researched, but their discussion is beyond the scope of this book. The two approaches discussed were developed by Cox and Vargas (1966) and Brennan (1972).

### Cox-Vargas Difference Index

The goal of criterion-referenced instruction is to bring each student to mastery without regard for group comparisons; criterion-referenced tests relate a student's performance to an a priori criterion. Consequently, a difficulty index is inappropriate, since, ideally, many items should be successfully completed by all students. The discrimination index may have some value for criterion-referenced tests, since a negative discrimination index is undesirable.

Cox and Vargas (1966) suggest a discrimination index determined by the difference between pretest and posttest difficulty based on answers from the same students to the same item before and after instruction. The resultant index is called a "difference index." An item with a difference index that does not increase from the pretest to the posttest is suspect. Like negatively discriminating items on norm-referenced examinations, items whose indices indicate a decrease in the number of students answering correctly from the pretest to the posttest are also viewed suspiciously.

The procedure and formulas for calculating the Cox-Vargas Difference Index follow:

1. Calculate pretest value:

$$\text{Pretest value} = \frac{\text{number of correct responses by item}}{N}$$

where $N$ is the total number of students in pretest group.

2. Calculate posttest value:

$$\text{Posttest value} = \frac{\text{number of correct responses by item}}{N}$$

where $N$ is the total number of students in posttest group.

3. Subtract the pretest value from the posttest value, and multiply the difference by 100:

$$DI = (\text{posttest value} - \text{pretest value}) \times 100$$

where $DI$ is the difference index.

### Example

An item on a classroom test is answered correctly by 25 of the 50 students who attempted it on the pretest. On the posttest, the same item is answered correctly by 40 of the 50 students who attempted to answer it. The difference index is calculated in the following manner:

$$DI = (\text{posttest value} - \text{pretest value}) \times 100$$
$$DI = \left(\frac{40}{50}\right) - \left(\frac{25}{50}\right) \times 100$$
$$DI = (0.8 - 0.5) \times 100$$
$$DI = (0.3) \times 100$$
$$DI = 30$$

A difference index of 30 indicates that the test item is measuring the intended learning. That is, 30% more students answered the item correctly in the posttest.

## Brennan's Index

A second approach was developed by Brennan (1972) and is referred to as the Brennan Index. This approach is also based on pretest and posttest scores; however, the major difference between the Cox-Vargas Difference Index and the Brennan Index is that the Cox-Vargas index is based on pretests and posttests of the same group, whereas Brennan identifies instructed and uninstructed groups. The latter may correspond to either pretest and posttest measures of the same group, or they may be two independent groups, one receiving instruction and one receiving no instruction.

The formula for the Brennan Index is as follows:

$$B = \left(\frac{N_{\text{right}}}{N_1}\right) - \left(\frac{N_{\text{wrong}}}{N_2}\right)$$

where $B$ is the Brennan Index, $N_1$ is the number of students in the instructed group, $N_2$ is the number of students in the uninstructed group, $N_{right}$ is the number of students in $N_1$ who got the item correct, and $N_{wrong}$ is the number of students in $N_2$ who got the item correct.

### Example

An item on a classroom test is answered correctly by 30 students in the instructed group and five students in the uninstructed group. There were 35 students in the instructed group and 30 students in the uninstructed group. The Brennan Index is found in the following way:

$$B = \left(\frac{N_{\text{right}}}{N_1}\right) - \left(\frac{N_{\text{wrong}}}{N_2}\right)$$

$$B = \left(\frac{30}{35}\right) - \left(\frac{5}{30}\right)$$

$$B = 0.86 - 0.17$$

$$B = +0.69$$

A greater percentage of students in the instructed group answered the item correctly. That is, 69% more students in the instructed group got the item correct.

To summarize, both Cox-Vargas (1966) and Brennan (1972) have developed difference indices; both require administration of the same examination before and after instruction. Both indices help identify poor test items. However, unlike a discrimination index based on low and high scorers, their indices "discriminate" between instructed and uninstructed learners. Items that fall below 0.50 in either index should be revised or replaced. A beneficial side-effect occurs when we calculate item analysis based on criterion-referenced examinations. After administering a pretest, the instructor has pretest scores to use for assessing previous learning and for planning future instruction.

## SUMMARY

Item analysis focuses on evaluation of an assessment instrument by examining the strengths and weaknesses of each individual test item. Item analysis can improve the assessment instrument, facilitate learning, improve teaching effectiveness, provide statistical information, and increase instructor skill in test construction.

Item analysis procedures focus on two basic statistical indices: a difficulty, or "easiness," index and a discrimination index. The difficulty index is the percentage of students tested who answer the item correctly. The discrimination index is a measure of how well an item discriminates between high achievers and low achievers on the total test.

The test item file serves as a permanent record for organizing the information resulting from an item analysis.

Item analysis procedures may have some limitations: (1) When class sizes are small, item analysis data are likely to be distorted. (2) If an item is deleted because of a poor discrimination index, the content validity of the test may be reduced. (3) It is extremely difficult to apply item analysis techniques to essay tests. (4) Item analysis techniques for criterion-referenced examinations are in their infancy.

By evaluating each test item, instructors can successfully monitor their assessment instruments, thus improving the quality of their examinations.

### REFERENCES

Ahmann, S. J., and Glock, M. D.: Evaluating pupil growth, ed. 4, Boston, 1971, Allyn and Bacon.

Brennan, R. L.: A generalized upper-lower item discrimination index, Educational and Psychological Measurement **32**: 289-303, 1972.

Cox, R. C., and Vargas, J. S.: A comparison of item selection techniques for norm-referenced and criterion-referenced tests (paper presented at the annual meeting of the National Council on Measurement in Education, Chicago, Ill., February 1966) ERIC Microfilms ED010517, 1966.

Crehan, K. D.: Item analysis for teacher-made mastery tests, Journal of Educational Measurement **11**(4):255-262, Winter 1974.

Lindquist, E. F., editor: Educational measurement, Washington, D.C., 1951, American Council on Education (fifth printing, Menasha, Wis., 1963, George Banta).

Popham, W. J., and Husek, T. R.: Implications of criterion-referenced measurement, Journal of Educational Measurement **6** (1): 1-9, 1969.

Scriven, M.: The methodology of evaluation, American Educational Research Association Monograph Series on Curriculum Evaluation, no. 1, 1967, pp. 39-83.

# 7

# Psychosocial concerns for testing

Explaining how the classroom instructor influences the behavior of students is difficult. Often the class has failed to perform because the instructor has failed to provide the kind of classroom environment that permits and encourages students to motivate themselves. In a well-managed classroom, students may produce several times as much work as they do in a less well-managed classroom. The most productive student may produce several times as much as the least productive student. How do we explain these wide variations in performance? How can instructors behave to promote more effective performance? In what ways can we encourage students to become self-motivated learners?

This chapter presents a plan for increasing student motivation. It describes the basic units of motivation as discussed by behaviorists. By blending this world of psychological thought with their personal instructional styles, instructors can help create a classroom environment that is both productive and personally satisfying.

## BEHAVIORIST APPROACH

The instructor controls the learning environment, the course assignments, and the consequences of classroom and clinical performance. By carefully controlling these three areas, the instructor can create a classroom environment that encourages high productivity and high student morale.

The interrelationships between the classroom and clinical environment, the classroom and clinical assignments, and the consequences of classroom and clinical performance are known by behaviorists as the "contingencies of reinforcement." The reward that is contingent on performance serves as a motivator for future performance. Whether instructors are aware of it or not, they are constantly shaping the behavior of their students by the way they utilize the rewards at their disposal. If carefully and properly applied by instructors, reinforcement theory can help increase their instructional effectiveness.

To adequately understand how reinforcement theory works, we must first understand some basic concepts relative to the theory. The necessary basic concepts are discussed in the following sections.

## Positive reinforcement

If a stimulus increases the probability of a response occurring when it is *added* to a situation, it is called "positive reinforcement" (Skinner, 1969). Behavior that leads to positive consequences tends to be repeated. It is extremely important to note that the behavior may or may not be seen by others as "good." However, if it is rewarded, the behavior will be continued. For example, if a student is consistently rewarded by the instructor for being uncooperative with the clinical staff, the student will continue to be uncooperative.

## Negative reinforcement

If a stimulus increases the probability of a response occurring when it is *removed* from the situation, it is called "negative reinforcement" (Skinner, 1969). This is sometimes referred to as "escape conditioning": the removal or avoidance of a noxious stimulus as a consequence of the performance of a response. For example, during a clinical rotation in obstetric nursing, a student may intensely dislike working in labor and delivery but enjoy the challenge of the newborn nursery. Consequently, the student is given the "unpleasant" task assignment (that is, labor and delivery) with the promise that when the assignment is completed the student can move to the more rewarding task (care of newborn).

## Extinction

The withholding of reinforcement following a response is called "extinction" (Skinner, 1969). After repeated nonreinforcement, the behavior decreases and will eventually disappear. The extinction principle may be used unthinkingly and eliminate desirable behavior. For example, a student announced to her peers at coffee that she had had it with good laboratory performance. For three weeks she had actively volunteered to participate in classroom discussions. What did it get her? Nothing, not one word of praise! Consequently, her solution was to stop talking. By withholding verbal reinforcement, the instructor had decreased student involvement in the learning process and harmed the student's morale.

In contrast, the extinction principle can be applied to eliminate undesirable behavior. For example, Instructor A was unknowingly reinforcing Rebecca's complaints of various maladies by listening attentively and offering suggestions for possible relief. In contrast, Instructor B ignored all complaints. As a result, Rebecca increased her complaining behavior to Instructor A and completely stopped complaining to Instructor B. Instructor B had effectively used extinction to stop Rebecca's complaining, whereas Instructor A was unconsciously increasing the complaining behavior.

## Punishment

If a noxious stimulus is presented in an attempt to eliminate an undesirable behavior, the process is called "punishment." The most controversial method for changing behavior, it has serious and undesirable emotional side-effects.

The fact that previously neutral people and objects can elicit feelings of well-being or feelings of intense stress is of immense practical importance. In classroom and clinical learning, this means that one can never teach a new knowledge or skill without simultaneously connecting some emotion or feeling to the knowledge or skill. The question is not whether there is an emotional effect, but whether the effect is positive or negative.

Consider a new student in psychiatric nursing who is expected to consistently offer therapeutic responses but finds adequate responses frustrating and difficult. If the clinical instructor ridicules her or generally makes the clinical environment punitive, the student will be conditioned to have negative feelings toward her psychiatric clinical experience. Later on, this "conditioning" may show up in her clinical performance evaluation as an assessment of *poorly motivated, undisciplined, hostile,* or *uncooperative.* For this student, learning to give therapeutic responses cannot be called an intellectual activity; her conditioned responses have interfered seriously with her intellectual activity.

Punishment may have several unexpected outcomes. Research provides sufficient evidence that reprimands intended as a mild form of punishment to stop certain behaviors may actually increase the frequency of those behaviors (Skinner, 1969).

Moderate punishment may suppress the unacceptable behavior but fail to produce a permanent change. For example, after receiving a speeding ticket on Main Street, a driver may stop speeding when on Main but speed on all other streets. Or, if a nurse is reprimanded for poor sterile technique, she may use sterile technique only when the punisher is in the area. At all other times, she may not adhere to sterile technique.

In contrast to mild or moderate punishment, extreme punishment is often accompanied by a wide variety of emotional side-effects. Long-term exposure to extreme punishment may lead to hypertension, ulcers, impairment of technical skills, and alienation.

In reality, punishment does not really eliminate an undesirable behavior; it only temporarily suppresses it. Furthermore, it leads to the avoidance of the punisher as well as of associated objects. More important, it does not work if used alone. The behavior usually emerges at a later time, stronger than ever. Certainly, pleasure is more successful in *increasing* responses than is pain or embarrassment in *decreasing* responses.

In light of the bleak picture of the effects of punishment, it would be nice to be able to conclude that instructors should never use punishment. Ideally, they should use extinction as the primary means of eliminating undesirable behavior. However, they may often use mild reprimands because extinction does not work fast enough to be effective.

For example, Janet was developing into a highly skilled cardiac nurse. She had mastered much of the prerequisite cognitive knowledge and psychomotor skills. However, she often spoke sharply to patients. By the time the instructor could reduce the rate of such behavior through extinction, many patients would be antagonized and unprofessionally treated. At the same time, punishment might have merely had the effect of reducing Janet's speaking sharply as long as the clinical instructor was present.

A recommended and practical solution to the problem is to teach Janet more appropriate staff/patient behaviors. If Janet speaks sharply, she should be immediately reprimanded; however, examples of good staff/patient communication should be introduced at the same time. When Janet displays good staff/patient behaviors, she should be praised immediately. That is, a contingency is introduced, and the correct response is rewarded by praise.

Punishment used in connection with positive reinforcement of the desirable response is much more effective in eliminating undesirable behavior than the use of either punishment, extinction, or reinforcement *alone*.

## Tips for using positive reinforcement
### Individualizing the reinforcers

The most important point in the selection of a reinforcer is to take care to select reinforcers that are seen as reinforcers for each individual. For example, learning a new clinical procedure may be more reinforcing for Karen than having increased patient contact; for Sarah, the reverse may be true. In another case, Marie may view the added responsibility of difficult patients as punitive, whereas Irene may view the assignment as a professional challenge.

### Making sure the rewards are distributed discriminately

The student must see a link between classroom or clinical performance and reward. Furthermore, the instructor must not give the same reward to all. The instructor must be willing to discriminate among students; otherwise the effectiveness is small. Students will compare their rewards with the rewards of their peers. Instructors who reward everyone at the same level merely encourage average performance (Deci, 1976). That is, superior performance is being extinguished while average performance is being strengthened. Furthermore, every student has a right to know if he or she is doing a good job.

### Letting students know the behaviors that will be rewarded

By clearly stating course objectives and the methods and procedures for evaluation, instructors can let students know what will be rewarded. If the desired behaviors are unclear or unrealistic in terms of available time and resources, the students will eventually become discouraged and stop trying. When the instructor makes the reward system clear, the students have a standard to measure themselves against.

### Letting students know what they are doing wrong

A student must have adequate and accurate information about his or her performance. Giving false assurance to an unsatisfactory student has dangerous long-term consequences. No one finds failure rewarding. By correcting undesirable behaviors and illustrating models of the desired behavior while using positive reinforcement, instructors can change student behavior without causing serious emotional side-effects.

### Positive reinforcers in the clinical setting

Four elements, or stages, constitute a clinically designed reinforcement program. They are represented schematically in Fig. 7-1 and briefly discussed below.

### Defining the desired classroom or clinical performance

A nursing instructor should clearly identify learning objectives for students. Without clearly defined objectives, teaching becomes disorganized, and students cannot separate the relevant information from the irrelevant information. The effectiveness of even the best teaching

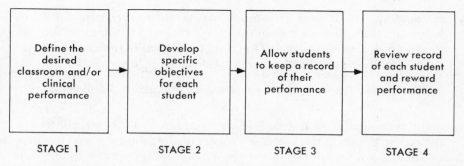

| Define the desired classroom and/or clinical performance | Develop specific objectives for each student | Allow students to keep a record of their performance | Review record of each student and reward performance |
|---|---|---|---|
| STAGE 1 | STAGE 2 | STAGE 3 | STAGE 4 |

**Fig. 7-1.** Elements of a clinically designed reinforcement program. (Adapted from Hamner, W. C., and Hamner, E. P.: Organizational Dynamics 4(4):3-21, Spring 1976.

is diminished if students are not aware of the purpose or do not understand what is expected of them. Once the behavioral aspects of the required learning are defined, the task of convincing students that learning is possible is simplified.

### Developing specific objectives for each student

Failure in individualizing objectives for students is often a major reason why instruction fails. To treat all students as though they were the same is to ignore the genetic, environmental, and motivational differences that exist among us. The fact that students learn at varying rates should be understood by instructors.

The approach to selecting specific objectives for each student that generally leads to the greatest acceptance is to allow the students to work closely with the instructor in setting objectives. The use of participatory classroom management techniques to enlist the ideas of the students results in the acceptance of the objectives and also stimulates students to come up with new objectives.

When setting objectives, instructors should consider that most people prefer to work toward objectives that are *moderately* difficult to attain rather than objectives that are *very* difficult to attain. Very difficult objectives have the highest reward value, but they are not as likely to be completed. In contrast, moderately difficult objectives have fairly high reward value with reasonable probability of completion; consequently, they are preferred.

### Allowing students to keep a written record of their performance

Student record keeping is called "self-feedback" and results in intrinsic rewards, or reinforcement from the task itself. Intrinsic rewards are powerful motivators. If a student has set an objective that involves learning a new clinical procedure, be prepared for a drop in the student's clinical performance. This drop in clinical performance is only temporary, however, because motivation remains high.

### Reviewing record of each student and rewarding performance

A crucial step in the program is the review of the student's record and the rewarding of the student's performance. This step allows the instructor to praise the positive aspects of the student's performance while withholding praise for below-average performance. Since each student has already recorded his or her own performance and knows the areas of deficiency, there is no good reason for the instructor to criticize the student. Negative criticism is self-induced, whereas praise comes from both the student and the instructor. This helps eliminate the emotional side-effects of criticism.

Traditional approaches to rewarding performance have concentrated on extrinsic, rather than intrinsic, rewards. Grades, release from a final, and scholarship money are examples of extrinsic rewards given to students. The focus on internal rewards is called "intrinsic motivation." Instead of an external reward, the reward is internal to the students and includes how they feel about themselves. Each student needs to feel effective or competent in relation to the classroom and clinical environment. This basic human need is the essence of intrinsic motivation (Deci, 1976). The growth, or intrinsic motivation, factors that are common to the nursing environment are *need for achievement, recognition of achievement, satisfaction in the work itself, responsibility,* and *the opportunity for personal growth.* Intrinsic rewards are powerful motivators.

Students often decide what to do based on their perceptions of which behaviors will lead to the most satisfaction. Sometimes a student will be seeking an extrinsic reward such as scholarship money, whereas at other times the need for achievement is primary. However, the message for instructors is that their students will decide how they will perform based on their expectations of the rewards that will follow.

To attract and keep good nursing students, it is necessary to satisfy personal needs. For example, students must be provided adequate classroom and clinical space, reasonable recreational facilities, and good library facilities. However, students also need personal achievement, recognition of achievement, professional growth, and advancement.

A classroom environment that is warm and rewarding, one in

which a student's accomplishments are met with recognition and praise, will be an environment of high productivity and student morale. Rather than fearing a behaviorist plot to change attitudes against the student's will, instructors need to understand that the behaviors desired in students must receive emphasis. Instead of hearing this: "I've had four different teachers and not one has even taken the trouble to see me as a human being. I'm just a machine and the only time I'm noticed is when I malfunction." Wouldn't it be better to hear this? "I don't mind being told when I've flubbed one as long as I'm told when I'm doing well."

## TEST ANXIETY

Freud formalized the concept of anxiety as a psychological construct. Manifestations include both physiological responses (such as palm sweating and increased pulse) and affective responses (such as feelings of uneasiness). Testing seems to arouse anxiety states in some students some of the time. Nursing educators are continually being exposed to students who verbalize their feelings of anxiety associated with testing. However, it was not until means were developed to measure test anxiety (Alpert and Haber, 1960, Sarason and others, 1958) that researchers could document the effects of test anxiety or could design methods of treatment for test anxiety.

Recent studies show that a statistically significant negative correlation exists between scores on test anxiety and scores on other tests: that is, as test anxiety scores increase, cognitive test scores decrease. Although the negative correlations do not indicate a direct causal relationship, they do provide clues to the effects of test anxiety.

Sarason and Hermatz (1965) found that highly test-anxious students did their best work under neutral appeal for achievement. What do these conclusions mean for the nurse educator? Often, when testing, the nursing instructor will advise the students to do their best work, suggesting that successful completion of the examination will prepare them for the clinical experience. The research findings seem to suggest that this may be a detrimental approach for highly test-anxious students.

In contrast, some nursing instructors attempt to put students at ease with expressions of approval. This also may be detrimental to the performance of highly test-anxious students. The research findings seem to suggest that *no advice* is best for such students.

Similarly, Wrightsman (1962) indicates that a stressful situation interferes with the successful performance of a complex task by highly anxious students. The performance of extremely anxious students in his study was decreased by almost one standard deviation by the increased stress of complicated instructions. In contrast, the test performance of the less anxious students was unchanged by the increased stress of complicated instructions. Consequently, one could conclude that the actual test performance of extremely anxious students may be affected by test instructions and that the actual test performance of the highly test-anxious student is not a valid indicator of achievement.

Some of the techniques that have been successful in decreasing test anxiety and increasing test scores are summarized below.

### Reduction of test anxiety through cognitive restructuring
(Goldfried, Linehan, and Smith, 1978)

Students in one research group were taught to put their unrealistic concerns and worries into a more realistic perspective, following the systematic, rational restructuring procedure outlined by Goldfried and Davison (1976).

During each session three situations were presented. Students were instructed to imagine themselves in the situation and to attempt to reduce their anxiety by means of rational restructuring. Immediately after a situation was presented, students were instructed (1) to record their self-defeating thoughts ("I can't learn this stuff; I'll probably fail; everyone's going to think I'm dumb"); (2) to record their rational reevaluation ("I may not fail; even if I do, I can retake the course; I really understand the material, why should I fail?"); and (3) to record their anxiety levels before and after reevaluation. A brief group discussion followed. Students were instructed to practice their reevaluation skills and were provided homework sheets with discussion material for the following session.

The study revealed that students in the systematic, rational restructuring group experienced greater anxiety reduction, whereas students in the control group did not change.

### Reduction of anxiety through self-controlled systematic desensitization (Spiegler and associates, 1976)

Self-controlled systematic desensitization involves actively teaching the student the skill of deep-muscle relaxation, which can be used to reduce feelings of anxiety whenever they occur. A major advantage of the self-control paradigm is that part of the treatment occurs outside the therapy sessions, in the real (not only the imagined) anxiety-provoking situations. Self-controlled desensitization involves training in the skill of deep-muscle relaxation that is not only useful in the setting or settings for which it is taught but also transferable to other anxiety-producing situations. The self-control conditioning leads to a reduction in self-reported test anxiety. On the test anxiety scale, self-control subjects report less anxiety about tests and studying. Similarly, on the stress measure students report greater reduction of anxiety. Lent and Russell (1978) have also found decreased test anxiety when systematic desensitization is incorporated into a study-skills training program.

### Reduction of test anxiety through the self-disclosing model (Sarason, 1975)

Highly test-anxious students were exposed to models who exhibited the following coping behaviors: (1) *coping anxious model* (model admitted to experiencing test anxiety but described methods of coping), (2) *noncoping anxious model* (model admitted to experiencing test anxiety but offered no way to cope with it), (3) *low-anxious model* (model admitted to being unworried about taking tests), and a (4) *neutral model* (model talked about campus life). The results indicated that, for highly test-anxious students, observation of the coping anxious model was most effective in reducing test anxiety; this would indicate that the self-disclosures provide the students with modeled information about adaptive behavior. A believable coping model may offer a convenient means of increasing stress tolerance and decreasing test anxiety.

Why do the other model conditions fail to decrease test anxiety? The noncoping model may remind highly anxious students of themselves, and the low-anxious model may not be credible to them. These interpretations may or may not be true, but they do suggest the value of observational learning.

### Reduction of test anxiety through group counseling and behavior therapy (Katahn, Strenger, and Cherry, 1966)

Highly test-anxious students were seen in a combination of group counseling and behavior therapy (systematic desensitization). Systematic desensitization was originally conceived as a passive, counterconditioning process to reduce anxiety. The client is taught a response that is incompatible with anxiety—often deep-muscle relaxation (Wolpe, 1958). While deeply relaxed, the client visualizes anxiety-producing situations, thereby conditioning the relaxation response to the anxiety-provoking situation. Grade point averages for the treated students showed a significant increase and Test Anxiety Scale scores showed a significant decrease after completion of the program. However, although students felt that the relaxation training was helpful, they all considered the group discussion to have played a more significant role in the reduction of their anxiety and the increase in their grade point averages.

Whereas the methods of coping with test anxiety emphasize the role of experimental approaches to decreasing test anxiety, an increased understanding of the underlying causes of the anxiety is important. Phillips, Martin, and Meyers (1972) have reported that socioeconomic differences in test anxiety have been discussed by many researchers. Higher levels of test anxiety reported by students with lower socioeconomic backgrounds may be related to several variables (such as low expectations of success, specific cognitive deficiencies, and lack of study skills). Additional research that would measure the effects of these related variables is needed to explore the relationship between socioeconomic status and test anxiety.

## SUMMARY

Creating a classroom environment that is both productive and personally satisfying is a goal of most educators. Often our favorite subject was favorite because of an instructor who reinforced our desire to learn by providing assistance, showing a personal interest, and respecting our opinions even though he or she didn't always agree with them.

In contrast, our least favored subject often achieved that status as the result of an instructor who humiliated and embarrassed us by threatening failure or highlighting our weaknesses in front of the class. The instructor who provides experiences with a high chance of success and offers appropriate praise will have a classroom environment with high productivity and high student morale.

Test anxiety is a common student complaint. Some of the techniques that have been used with success to decrease test anxiety are (1) cognitive restructuring, (2) self-controlled systematic desensitization, (3) self-disclosing models, and (4) group counseling and behavior therapy.

### REFERENCES

Alpert, R., and Haber, R. N.: Anxiety in academic achievement situations, Journal of Abnormal and Social Psychology **61**:207-215, 1960.

Deci, E. L.: The hidden costs of rewards, Organizational dynamics **4** (3):61-72, Winter 1976.

Goldfried, M. R., and Davison, G. C.: Clinical behavior therapy, New York, 1976, Holt, Rinehart & Winston, Inc.

Goldfried, M. R., Linehan, M., and Smith, J.: Reduction of test anxiety through cognitive restructuring, Journal of Consulting and Clinical Psychology **46**(1):32-39, 1978.

Hamner, W. C., and Hamner, E. P.: Behavior modification on the bottom line, Organizational Dynamics 4(4):3-21, Spring 1976.

Herzberg, F.: One more time; how do you motivate employees? Harvard Business Review **46**(1):53-62, January-February 1968.

Katahn, M., Strenger, S., and Cherry, N.: Group counseling and behavior therapy with test-anxious college students, Journal of Consulting Psychology **30**(6):544-549, 1966.

Lent, R. W., and Russell, R. K.: Treatment of test anxiety by cue-controlled de-sensitization and study-skills training, Journal of Counseling Psychology **25**(3):217-224, 1978.

Phillips, B. N., Martin, R. P., and Meyers, J.: School-related interventions with anxious children. In Spielberger, C. D., editor: Anxiety; current trends in theory and research, vol. 2, New York, 1972, Academic Press, Inc.

Sarason, I. G.: Test anxiety and the self-disclosing coping model, Journal of Consulting and Clinical Psychology **43**(2):148-153, 1975.

Sarason, S., and Hermatz, M. C.: Test anxiety and experimental conditions, Journal of Personality and Social Psychology **1**:499-505, 1965.

Sarason, S., and others: A test anxiety scale for children, Child Development **29**:105-113, 1958.

Skinner, B. F.: Contingencies of reinforcement, New York, 1969, Appleton-Century-Crofts.

Spiegler, M. D., and others: A self-control versus a counter conditioning paradigm for systematic de-sensitization; an experimental comparison, Journal of Counseling Psychology **23**(1):83-86, 1976.

Wolpe, J.: Psychotherapy by reciprocal inhibition, Stanford, Calif., 1958, Stanford University Press.

Wrightsman, L. S.: The effects of anxiety, achievement motivation and task importance on intelligence test performance, Journal of Educational Psychology **53**:150-156, 1962.

# 8

# Grading

Grades, unfortunately, are a major concern of students and faculty. It is not unusual for students to be more concerned with the grade they receive in community health than with the knowledge, skills, and attitudes they learn from taking the course. Obviously, this is a misplacement of priorities. Grades are often criticized and opposed for this and other reasons. They are sometimes used unwisely, misinterpreted, overinterpreted, or handled as weapons rather than as one of many sources of information (Ebel, 1972). Neither the grades we give nor the uses to which they have been put are beyond criticism.

Some nursing instructors increasingly believe that in many, if not all, instructional situations a criterion-referenced (pass/fail) system of grading is the most humane and effective method of evaluating students. Others have a strong preference for a systematic comparison of the performance of individuals with that of their peers (norm-referenced grading). Furthermore, some nursing instructors believe that grades should be used to reward students for growth as well as for final achievement.

This chapter focuses on two major dilemmas in grading: (1) norm-referenced versus criterion-referenced grades and (2) grades based on growth versus grades based on final achievement. Problems inherent in weighing grades and the current phenomenon of grade inflation are also discussed.

## NORM-REFERENCED GRADES

Norm-referenced grading and testing involve sampling of the entire domain of skills, knowledges, and attitudes that define the instructional unit. This sampling may include performances clearly above as well as below the level an instructor may wish to set as a minimum level of proficiency.

# Functions served by norm-referenced grades
## *Provide students with information to guide their present learning*

Regular monitoring of student progress provides students with the psychological security of knowing where they stand in relation to the class and in relation to the objectives of the course. It also facilitates learning in a more direct and controlled way.

Instructors should inform their students in advance of the administration of any tests, quizzes, or other monitoring instruments. Surprise quizzes based on the rationale that mature students should always be up-to-date and continuously studying do not always keep the students up-to-date. However, surprise examinations do cause and maintain an unnecessary level of test anxiety, which is not recommended for effective learning. Furthermore, once a test has been given, it is important to report the results to the students as soon as possible. Immediate feedback facilitates learning and helps to maintain optimum levels of motivation.

## *Provide one of the best predictors of future grades* (Hoyt and Munday, 1966)

Norm-referenced grades play an important role in informing both the student and the academic institution of prospects for the student's academic success. As a result, norm-referenced grades in the form of grade point averages play an important role in admission to nursing programs. Some educators oppose this practice and appeal for the additional use of other types of data, such as the personal interview, related volunteer work experience, and letters of recommendation. Currently there is much controversy and discussion about this matter. Mann (1977) completed a dissertation on the reliability of interviews for predicting success in the health professions. His study is a serious attempt to go beyond grades as the primary criteria for admissions selection. Obviously, data in addition to grades are critical when 300 students meet a minimum grade point average requirement and only 50 students can be selected.

## *Provide important information for program evaluation*

Most nursing programs are required to record Nursing Board Examination scores and other descriptors of program achievement. This record of performance is useful to administrators as they compare and contrast the effectiveness and efficiency of the program from year to year. In addition, this information may be used to prepare recommendations for graduates seeking employment or further education.

If only 55% of a program's students pass the registration examination, we might conclude that the program is not very effective. In addition, if the per-student costs for the program are high, we might question its efficiency. However, the program could be both fairly ineffective and inefficient and still be essential to the state's nursing supply. If this were the case, more in-depth review, possibly coupled with additional finances and faculty, would be required to improve the program.

Educators must also recognize the serious gap between state board test items and dynamic, futuristic nursing programs. When the nursing program is teaching and testing concepts and principles above and beyond those tested by state board examinations, these state board scores are obviously not reflective of the student's present achievement or future performance and potential. For example, the theoretical dimensions of professional bureaucratic work conflicts may be explored in class through an analysis of work tasks and organizational theory. However, state board examinations would not reflect the student's knowledge in this area.

### Provide a mechanism to determine teaching effectiveness

Student success on licensing, registry, and certifying examinations is strong evidence of effective teaching. It is important to remember, however, that this information must be viewed in light of other relevant factors, such as length of clinical experience, availability of remedial education, student characteristics, and age of the program.

No attempt should be made to openly compare individual faculty with select portions of the licensing or certifying examinations. Such practices will foster rivalry and decrease professional cooperation between nursing instructors. If this professional cooperation were lost, it could eventually lead to poorly prepared graduates and a weaker nursing program.

### Provide faculty with diagnostic evaluation to focus instruction by determining a starting point

Diagnostic testing before instruction helps the instructor determine a starting point for instruction. For example, if nursing students were not yet familiar with the concept of antigens and antibodies, it would be difficult to discuss Rh incompatibility in the obstetric nursing unit.

If diagnostic testing is done before admission to a nursing program, serious consideration should be given to the results of verbal skill scores. Research has shown that the degree to which a student's poor verbal skills can be altered is inversely related to the age at which remediation begins. Only the most powerful environmental conditions are likely to produce significant changes in later grades (Bloom, 1964). Consequently, remedial programs should be strong in the primary grades where they can be the most effective. This research has serious implications for nursing programs. If hopeful students have seriously weak verbal skills and are accepted into a collegiate program, they will probably experience frustration, hostility, and failure.

Another form of placement diagnosis involves assessment of the degree to which a student has already mastered course objectives. For example, college proficiency examinations allow students who have already achieved course objectives to receive course credit after successful completion of the examinations.

The instructor may also wish to use the final examination as a pretest. Some students may not display the required level of mastery on the pretest but still possess some of the competencies the course seeks to develop. If this is the case, the instructor may add enrichment units or otherwise change the course. Furthermore, if the instructor has broken the course into units and has built formative tests for each unit, these units may be used for more specific diagnosis. If formative tests are not available, the instructor may gain valuable information through a careful analysis of errors on the more traditional pretest.

## Advantages and limitations of norm-referenced grades

The primary advantages of norm-referenced grades are the following:

- They provide a summary of each student's relative performance in terms that are easily understood by students, instructors, and administrators.
- They provide a mechanism for ranking achievement (superior, above average, average, below average, failure).
- They help to identify the least able students so that remedial help can be provided to them.
- They determine entry and exit expectations.

The primary limitations of norm-referenced grades include the following:

- They may not specifically indicate how well a student has mastered an essential skill. For example, in a purely norm-referenced grading system, an A could be a score of 56% right and an F a score of 10% right. In fact, essentially everyone would have earned an F.
- They force many students to view themselves as failures or as among the lowest achievers in the class. Emotional problems

may result, or, at the very least, students may react with defensive behavior because of their fear of disapproval or failure.

## CRITERION-REFERENCED GRADES

Criterion-referenced grades indicate assessment of a skill, knowledge, or attitude against a series of performances that represent minimum levels of acceptable performance. Consequently, students do not generally compete with their peers; rather, they strive for an established criterion or competency in the skills, attitudes, and knowledge being tested.

To adequately discuss criterion-referenced grades, we should be familiar with the theory and practice of mastery learning. Mastery learning is the theoretical basis on which the concept of criterion-referenced grades was developed. Mastery learning is one of the most powerful ideas to shape educational views and practices (Block, 1971). It assumes that all, or almost all, students can learn and describes explicit procedures whereby most students can achieve at high levels. This concept is also the precursor of competency-based nursing instruction. In practice, mastery learning is often referred to as competency-based instruction, criterion-referenced instruction, or individualized instruction.

### History of mastery learning

The concept of mastery learning is not new. As early as the 1920's, there were at least two major attempts to produce mastery in students' learning: the first attempt was the Winnetka Plan developed by C. Washburne and his associates (1922); the second was an approach developed by H. C. Morrison (1932) at the University of Chicago. The two approaches shared the following features:

- Mastery was defined in terms of educational objectives.
- Instruction was organized into well-defined learning units. Each unit consisted of a collection of learning materials systematically arranged to teach the desired learning objectives.
- Mastery of each unit was required before a new unit could be taught.
- Ungraded diagnostic progress tests were administered at the completion of each unit.
- On the basis of the diagnostic test results, each student's original instruction was supplemented with appropriate learning experiences.

Some differences between the approaches are presented in Table 8-1.

Although mastery learning was popular into the 1930's, it all but

**Table 8-1.** Comparison of Washburne and Morrison mastery learning approaches

| Winnetka Plan (1922) | Morrison (1932) |
| --- | --- |
| 1. Objectives were cognitive. | 1. Objectives were cognitive, psychomotor, and affective. |
| 2. Teachers primarily used self-instructional materials. | 2. Teachers used a variety of instructional strategies (reteaching, tutoring, restructuring the learning activities). |
| 3. Each student was allowed all the time needed for mastery of a unit. | 3. Each student was allowed the time required to bring almost all students to unit mastery. |

disappeared for approximately 20 years. The concept reappeared in the late 1950's and early 1960's as an adjunct to programmed instruction. A basic tenet of programmed instruction is that learning any behavior, no matter how complex, rests on the learning of a sequence of less complex component behaviors. This learning principle was developed by Skinner (1954). He taught animals complex behaviors through "shaping" (also referred to as "successive approximations"). For example, Skinner (1951) used shaping to train a rat to perform the following behavioral sequence:

1. Pick up marble in first corner.
2. Transfer marble to second corner.
3. Return to center.
4. Go to third corner.
5. Pick up marble in second corner.
6. Bow in four directions.

The rat would be reinforced every time it moved in the desired direction. By reinforcing only successive approximations to the desired behavior, Skinner could teach the rat a complex behavioral repertoire. Skinner's primary concern was in discovering the relationship between the reinforcement and the behavior. The basic strength of Skinner's operant behaviorism and of shaping is that each is firmly rooted in a strong research base.

Programmed instruction is Skinner's application of this research to learning: learning is broken down into small tasks, and successful completion of each task is reinforced. Theoretically, this approach ensures learning of each task and makes it possible for each student to master complex tasks. Many educational psychologists believe that moving on to new material before prerequisite tasks have been mastered may be a primary failing of our educational system.

Programmed instruction seemed so promising that by the mid-1960's there were major attempts to develop entire curricula using this approach. It worked well for some students but not for all. As a result, programmed instruction did not provide a complete mastery learning model. However, it did contribute major concepts to learning theory.

Another significant overall learning model was developed by Carroll (1963) and expanded by Bloom (1976). The full Carroll model proposes that, under the typical learning conditions, the time spent in learning and the time needed are functions of certain student and instructional characteristics:

$$\text{Degree of learning} = f\left(\frac{\text{time actually spent}}{\text{time needed}}\right)$$

The time spent is determined by the amount of time allowed and the student's perseverance. Therefore, the model expanded is as follows:

$$\text{Degree of learning} = f\left(\frac{\text{time allowed, perseverance}}{\text{time needed}}\right)$$

The time needed for instruction is determined by the student's aptitude for the task, the quality of the instruction, and the student's ability to understand the instruction.

$$\text{Degree of learning} = f\left(\frac{\text{time allowed, perseverance}}{\substack{\text{aptitude, quality of instruction, student's ability} \\ \text{to understand the instruction}}}\right)$$

### Time allowed

Schools are organized to give group instruction with definite times allotted for particular learning tasks. Whatever the time allotted by the school and the curriculum, it is likely to be too much for some students and not enough for others.

Carroll (1963) believes the time spent on learning is the key to mastery. His basic assumption is that aptitude determines the rate of learning and that most, if not all, students can achieve mastery if they devote the amount of time needed to the learning. However, time alone does not ensure learning. Husén (1967) found a negative correlation between achievement test scores in mathematics and number of hours per week of homework in mathematics as reported by students. This would imply the amount of time spent on homework is not an indicator of mathematics achievement.

Many educational psychologists are convinced that it is not the sheer amount of time spent in learning that accounts for the level of learning. All students should be allowed the time they need to learn a subject. The time is likely to be affected by aptitude, verbal ability, quality of instruction, and quality of out-of-class help. The task of the instructor in mastery learning is to find ways of altering the time as well as the instruction to enhance learning (Bloom, Hastings, and Madaus, 1971).

### Perseverance

"Perseverance" is the time the learner is willing to spend on a task (Carroll, 1963). As students find the effort rewarding, they are likely to spend more time on a specific learning task. However, if completion of the task produces little or no success, the students may, in self-defense, decrease the amount of time devoted to the task. Although each individual's frustration level varies, all students will sooner or later stop trying if the task is too difficult and painful. Frequency of reward and evidence of success will increase the student's perseverance. As a student attains mastery in a given task, the student's perseverance in a related task is likely to increase.

### Aptitude

In study after study, it has been found that aptitude tests are relatively good predictors of achievement. However, this is true only if the aptitude and achievement measures are valid and reliable. For example, a good set of mathematics aptitude tests may have a correlation as high as +0.70 with the final grade in a unit on drug dosages and solutions.

The use of aptitude tests for predictive purposes and the high correlations between such tests and achievement criteria have led many educators to believe that high levels of achievement are only possible for the most able students (Bloom, Hastings, and Madaus, 1971).

In contrast to this is Carroll's view that *aptitude is the amount of time required by the learner to attain mastery of a learning task.* Implicit is the assumption that, given enough time, all students can conceivably attain mastery of a learning task. Carroll is convinced that the grade of A as an index of mastery of a subject can, under appropriate conditions, be achieved by 95% of the students in a class. He assumes that it will take some students more effort, time, and help to achieve this level than it will others. And there will be those for whom the effort and help required may be prohibitive.

A basic problem in development of a mastery learning strategy is to find ways of reducing the amount of time the slower students require to a point where it is not prohibitively long. It is this problem that must be directly attacked by strategies for mastery learning.

### Quality of instruction

The quality of instruction is the degree to which the presentation, explanation, and ordering of elements of the task to be learned approach the optimum for a given learner (Carroll, 1963). Some students learn quite well through independent study, whereas others need traditional lectures with concrete examples and verbal explanations. Some students need constant reinforcement and verbal approval; some may need spaced repetition of the course materials, whereas others understand after one explanation.

### Ability to understand instruction

In most college courses, there is a single teacher and a single set of instructional materials. If students find it easy to understand the teacher and the textbook, they have little difficulty in learning the subject. If they find it hard to understand the instruction, the material, or both, they are likely to have great difficulty learning the subject. Here is a point at which the students' abilities interact with the instructional materials and the instructor's skill in teaching. However, given help and various types of aids, individual teachers can find ways of modifying their instruction to fit the differing needs of their students.

In summary, Carroll proposes that if students are normally distributed with respect to aptitude but the kind and quality of instruction and the amount of time available for learning are made appropriate to the characteristics and needs of each student, the majority of students may be expected to achieve mastery of the subject.

Bloom (1968) transformed Carroll's conceptual model into a working model for mastery learning. Bloom hypothesized the following:

If aptitudes predict the rate at which, and not necessarily the level to which, a student can learn a task, then it should be possible to fix the degree of learning expected at some mastery level and to manipulate the instructional variables in Carroll's model so that almost all students meet mastery.

If students are normally distributed with respect to aptitude for a subject and are provided *uniform* instruction (in terms of quality and learning time), then student achievement will also be normally distributed.

However, if students are normally distributed in regard to aptitude but each student receives both optimal quality of instruction and sufficient time, most of the students can reach mastery. As a result, there is little or no relationship between aptitude and achievement. Consequently, aptitude is really still normally distributed, but achievement will be high for almost all learners.

Bloom proposed to implement these ideas in the typical classroom, where the time allowed for learning is relatively fixed. His mastery learning model has the following characteristics:

- Mastery is defined in terms of a specific set of objectives.
- The content is broken into small learning units (two weeks instruction per unit is suggested).
- The instructor teaches each unit with traditional instructional methods.
- Diagnostic tests are given at the end of each unit.
- Supplementary instruction is provided based on the results of the unit diagnostic test.

Martin (1977) tested this mastery model for four years, using 222 students enrolled in a human anatomy course. Five students dropped the course, one received an F, and two received B's. Achievement of the criterion established for mastery and the grade of A was accomplished by 214 students.

## Criterion-referenced tests

To develop a criterion-referenced test based on mastery learning concepts or reflective of a competency-based curriculum, the nursing instructor must complete the following steps:

1. State competencies to be demonstrated.
2. Determine the criteria that identify successful completion of the competency.
3. Provide for student demonstration of the stated competencies.

The check list shown in Table 8-2, for example, can be used to assess whether the student can determine and record vital signs.

It is easy to record *yes* or *no* (the student can or cannot read and record vital signs accurately) and on completion give a pass/fail or satisfactory/unsatisfactory grade. However, student demonstration of other competencies may be much harder to define. The rating scale shown in Table 8-3 could be used to assess whether a student successfully instructed a diabetic patient, but the observer would have more qualitative decisions to make. With a qualitative rating scale instead of a check list, the subjectiveness of the measurement increases. Whereas instructors can unequivocally state that all students have mastered taking vital signs, mastery of instructing the diabetic patient is much more subjective. Of course, a well-designed rating scale is an asset to any education assessment program.

**Table 8-2.** Check list for vital signs

| Performance | Yes | No | Comments |
|---|---|---|---|
| 1.0 Pulse<br>  1.1 Prepares patient<br>  1.2 Counts accurately<br>  1.3 Records accurately | | | |
| 2.0 Respiration<br>  2.1 Prepares patient<br>  2.2 Counts accurately<br>  2.3 Records accurately | | | |
| 3.0 Blood pressure<br>  3.1 Prepares patient<br>  3.2 Counts accurately<br>  3.3 Records accurately | | | |
| 4.0 Temperature<br>  4.1 Prepares patient<br>  4.2 Reads accurately<br>  4.3 Records accurately | | | |

**Table 8-3.** Rating scale for instruction of diabetic patients

SA, Strongly agree
A, Agree
U, Undecided
D, Disagree
SD, Strongly disagree

| Performance | SA | A | U | D | SD | Comments |
|---|---|---|---|---|---|---|
| 1. Student presented information to patient in an organized way. | | | | | | |
| 2. Student spoke slowly and clearly when explaining to the patient. | | | | | | |
| 3. Student gave accurate instructions. | | | | | | |
| 4. Student adjusted information to the educational background of the patient. | | | | | | |
| 5. Student demonstrated sensitivity to the patient's needs. | | | | | | |
| 6. Student followed hospital policies during the instruction. | | | | | | |
| 7. Student maintained a professional manner while instructing. | | | | | | |

Although the notion of mastery, or competency-based, instruction is appealling, it may be deceptive (Ebel, 1972). Complete mastery of any but the simplest skills and knowledge is often unattainable. For example, it is relatively easy to measure mastery of the lower cognitive levels (knowledge, comprehension, and application); however, the measurement of mastery of the higher cognitive levels (analysis, synthesis, and evaluation) is much more difficult. What we are actually reporting when we adopt a criterion-referenced grading system are the minimum skills and knowledge needed to measure the competency (Ebel, 1972).

## Advantages and limitations of criterion-referenced grades

The primary advantages of criterion-referenced grades are the following:

- They provide a measure of achievement tied solely to a student's ability to demonstrate specific knowledges and skills rather than to the student's rank among peers on a given quantitative measurement device.
- They generally emphasize minimum proficiency. All students who can perform at a minimum level of performance (criterion level) receive a passing grade. This often produces greater student interest in and a more positive attitude toward the subject.
- They generally do not force students to view themselves as failures or as among the lowest achievers in class. This is of tremendous psychological value. In contrast, frequent indications of failure are bound to be accompanied by increased self-doubt in the student.
- They decrease intergroup competition. Small-group study is encouraged without the danger of students' giving one another special advantages in a competitive situation. In addition to helping the slower students, the group process encourages abler students to strengthen their learning as they help others understand concepts through alternative explanations and applications.

The primary limitations of criterion-referenced grades are as follows:

- They may necessitate repeated testing to make sure that most students meet the criterion level of performance. This brings with it the additional problem of writing multiple, parallel test forms for use in repeated testing. Instructors find it difficult to write test items for as many as four possible tests per unit. Furthermore, some students are often embarrassed if they repeatedly fail the criterion-referenced tests.

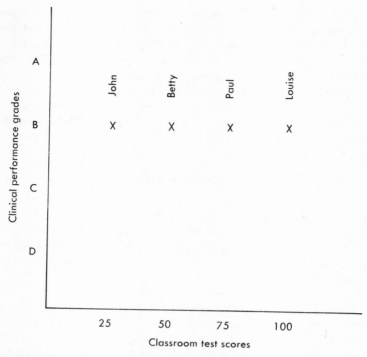

**Fig. 8-1.** Comparison between classroom and clinical performance.

- They allow some loss of valuable information when only two levels of achievement are reported (satisfactory/unsatisfactory or pass/fail). Did the student require one or five attempts to perform satisfactorily? In addition, when students perform slightly above the criterion, they are graded as completely satisfactory, whereas an achievement ever so slightly below is treated as unsatisfactory.

- They promote the misconception that by comparing a student's performance with some fixed standard, we negate the need to make comparisons between students.

- They require appropriate measures of reliability, just like other tests; however, the development of such measures remains in its infancy. Since criterion-referenced test scores only differentiate between minimum acceptable performance and unacceptable performance, there is little or no variation of scores on a variable. When this occurs, reliability coefficients become meaningless. If reliability is computed, it will approximate zero. For example,

Fig. 8-1 illustrates a scatter diagram representing comparisons between clinical performance grades based on pass/fail and classroom test scores. If a reliability measure were calculated to determine a consistency measurement for the clinical performance reported in Fig. 8-1, it would be meaningless since there is no variation of scores on that variable. When we try to compare the clinical performance with the classroom test scores reported in Fig. 8-1, we also get meaningless information.

Although mastery learning, with its resultant criterion-referenced testing and competency-based instruction, offers a utopian promise, it is not without critics. Many educators believe the tremendous expense in terms of time and effort outweighs its benefits. Some educators applying this learning strategy will fall far short of the mastery level identified. Some educators recommend criterion-referenced testing for the lower levels of cognitive learning only, protesting that when we try to develop criterion-referenced tests for the upper cognitive levels we get a high correlation between test results and the student's general intelligence.

Some critics claim there is arbitrariness in the definition of *mastery* and in the choice of specifics to master. Others believe there is the pedagogical danger of placing emphasis on specifics rather than on the theoretical basis of the instruction. Although there are many situations in nursing programs where criterion-referenced grades are more suitable than norm-referenced grades, the belief that criterion-referenced tests are generally superior is open to debate.

In summary, criterion-referenced grades only tell us if the student has reached minimum proficiency. They do not tell us the overall quality of the student's ability. However, they are excellent tools for measuring educational objectives that require a yes or no answer and for reporting on psychomotor or skill-related competencies.

## NONEDUCATIONAL CAUSES OF ACADEMIC FAILURE

Every instructor recognizes that a few students are properly placed but are still unsuccessful. For these students, changing instruction and materials still does not produce the expected level of learning. Noneducational causes of academic failure may be physical, psychological, or environmental. These categories often overlap. For example, environmental factors may trigger health problems that may result in psychological problems.

Marie, a very competent graduate student with a high Graduate Record Examination score and a 3.5 grade point average, was doing poorly in almost all areas of her graduate nursing program. When ad-

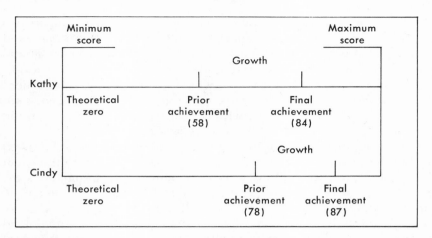

**Fig. 8-2.** Growth versus achievement in a pediatric nursing course. (Adapted from Ahmann, S. J., and Glock, M. D.: Evaluating pupil growth, Boston, 1971, Allyn & Bacon, Inc., p. 501.)

vising Marie, we discovered that she was a Mormon and strongly missed the contacts with the Mormon church and its resultant emotional support. In addition, she was in her early thirties and was using graduate school as a substitute for the home and children she hoped to have. After a year of graduate study, Marie left school two weeks before finals. No encouragement from the professional staff could change her mind.

Such noneducational causes of failure to learn are beyond the control of any instructor. We must constantly remember that the school may not be able to help some students who are suffering from physical, psychological, or environmental problems. No learning model is a panacea; there are too many variables beyond the instructor's control.

## GROWTH VERSUS ACHIEVEMENT

Final grades may report growth *or* achievement. These are distinct concepts. *Growth* means gain or change; *achievement* means present accomplishments. To measure growth reliably, we must have a discrete measure of the student's entering behavior (Ahmann and Glock, 1971). In contrast, to measure achievement we must compare the student's present performance with established norms and evaluate it without respect to the student's prior experiences. Fig. 8-2 illustrates the difference between grading based on growth and grading based on achievement.

Kathy enters pediatric nursing with a pretest score of 58; Cindy has a pretest score of 78. On entering, then, Cindy has a greater knowledge of pediatric nursing than does Kathy. However, final course grades indicate that Kathy received an overall average of 84 and Cindy received an overall average of 87. Both students have successfully mastered new course material. Although Kathy shows significant growth, Cindy's final course average is still greater.

The problem facing nursing instructors is truly a dilemma. How do we reward Kathy for her tremendous growth strides and encourage Cindy to grow more, especially when it is common knowledge that it is much more difficult to raise a high score even higher than to raise a low score.

The hard fact remains that we are preparing individuals to become competent nurses and our major concern should be: Can Kathy and Cindy function adequately as pediatric nurses? The need to prepare highly skilled health professionals dictates that all our students must be graded primarily on achievement. Of course, this does not negate our responsibility to provide psychological encouragement and remedial help.

When we pass our students in pediatric nursing, we are certifying to the next instructor that they have achieved the course objectives. We should not give fraudulent certification, since we would be doing a disservice to the student, the prospective employer, and, most important, the pediatric patient.

## WEIGHING ASSESSMENT DATA

Analysis of the course objectives usually suggests that certain activities, papers, and examinations will be the most appropriate tools for gathering evidence of the extent to which a student has achieved the course objectives. In nursing education, for example, examinations, interviews, check lists, rating scales, case studies, and anecdotal records are all used as indicators of achievement. These indicators must be combined in some way to report a single composite symbol of student performance. How should the weight for each component be determined?

Two important constructs can help determine the desirable effective weight for each assessment indicator. The first of these is the *validity* of the information. Does the case study measure the student's ability to problem solve? The second consideration is *reliability*. If the instructor regrades the case study, will the results remain consistent? These constructs—validity and reliability—should temper the weights that are assigned to each assessment tool (Thorndike and

Hagen, 1969). For all practical purposes, validity and reliability will be highest for carefully prepared objective tests and yes/no check lists. Validity and reliability will be moderate for essay tests, written papers, and rating scales and lowest for class participation and oral reports.

It should be noted that there is no easy mechanism for determining appropriate weights for grading purposes; however, the above suggestions are rational guidelines. Remember, it is truly impossible to remove all subjectivity from grades. Often the fine line between a B and C rests on the professional judgment of the instructor. Grading practices are expressions of individual and group value systems as much as they are dispassionate reports of student progress (Thorndike and Hagen, 1969).

## GRADE INFLATION

For the past decade there has been a growing concern with the steady improvement in scholastic performances of undergraduates as reflected by grade point averages. This index has consistently increased since 1963, from 2.49 to 2.94 in 1974 (Suslow, 1977). The phenomenon has been termed "grade inflation." It suggests that admissions counselors, instructors, and employers must somehow reinterpret the scholastic records of students.

There are several possible explanations for this trend. Many of the reasons for grade inflation are in part unmeasurable and speculative but, nevertheless, worthy of discussion.

Many colleges and universities have changed their traditional grading policies, adopting alternative grading systems—pass/fail, credit/no credit—and allowing course withdrawals without penalty up to two weeks before the final examination. These options have reduced the inclusion of poor or failing grades in students' records. At the State University of New York at Buffalo, the faculty senate is currently engaged in spirited discussions regarding grading policies, specifically the satisfactory/unsatisfactory (S/U) option. At present, faculty have little control over whether students opt for S/U. The faculty senators have recommended that the S/U option continue for up to 25% of each student's total credit hours, with the constraint that students on academic probation not be granted this option. Some instructors are arguing that, although the original intent of the S/U option was to encourage students to explore areas outside their major field without fear of academic penalty, many are using the option to avoid C's and D's. This issue still remains to be solved. However, it does illustrate a faculty attempt to help contain grade inflation.

A larger percentage of A grades are being awarded. A Carnegie survey of 25,000 undergraduates reports a far higher proportion of A's in 1975 than in 1969 (Trow, 1977). Furthermore, a national survey conducted at Berkeley shows that, since the mid-1960's the percentage of A grades has more than doubled, from 16% to 34%, while the percentage of C grades has been cut by almost half, from 37% to 21% (Suslow, 1977).

Many college instructors agree that the Vietnam War, accompanied by student unrest in the 1960's, also influenced grading practices. Many instructors were reluctant to give failing grades, because they knew that unless their students remained in college they were likely to be drafted to fight in an unpopular war. Perhaps as significant, there was also an increase in student activism demanding a voice on academic policies, including formulation of grading policy.

In addition, educational institutions are fighting to maintain their enrollments as the number of potential students diminishes. To maintain enrollment, passing grades are often given to students who would have previously failed. Similarly, average students are pressuring faculty for above-average grades because of their intense desire to enter graduate school.

The University of California at Berkeley has recommended two ways to help contain the rise in grades:

- Redesign transcripts to record the student's course grade, the average grade earned by others in the course, and the class size.
- Provide a complete list of undergraduate courses, including instructors' names and percentage distributions of letter grades A through F.

Obviously, these procedures would provide more information about the relative rigor of the grading programs to graduate programs, professional schools, and employers. However, they might not ensure a slowing of the rise in grades. Given instructors' strong belief in academic freedom, especially as it relates to grading practices, the mere publication of grade distributions may be ineffective in reducing grade inflation. In fact, the second option, that of publishing instructor names along with the grade distribution, may increase grade inflation by identifying "easy graders."

To increase the general confidence that grades are valid indicators of academic success, educational institutions must discuss and clarify their grading standards and policies.

## SUMMARY

Grades are a major concern of nursing educators as they try to document student achievement. Some prefer norm-referenced grading (a comparison of the performance of students with the performance of their peers). Others prefer criterion-referenced grading, based on mastery learning concepts.

Norm-referenced grades (1) provide students with information to guide their present learning, (2) are one of the best predictors of future grades, (3) provide essential information for program evaluation, (4) provide a mechanism for determining teaching effectiveness, and (5) supply faculty with diagnostic evaluation to focus instruction by determining a starting point.

Criterion-referenced grades provide a measure of achievement related solely to a student's ability to demonstrate specific knowledges and skills. Mastery learning provides the theoretical basis on which the concept of criterion-referenced grades was developed. A mastery learning model proposes that the time spent in learning and time needed for learning are functions of student and instructional characteristics.

When we finally grade students, we are certifying to the next instructor that they have achieved the course objectives. We should not give fraudulent certification. Although the measurement of growth is desirable, grading based on achievement is essential to preparing competent nursing professionals.

There is no easy mechanism for weighing student grades. However, validity and reliability are highest for objective tests and yes/no check lists; moderate for essay tests, written reports, and rating scales; and lowest for class participation and oral reports.

Grade inflation, that is, the steady increase in grade point averages, has been documented. This phenomenon suggests that admissions counselors, instructors, and employers must somehow reinterpret the scholastic records of students.

To summarize student performance by transforming objective and subjective data into a symbol that measures achievement is extremely difficult. With increased teaching experience and increased knowledge in the area of tests and measurement, nursing instructors can make sound judgments with greater consistency.

**REFERENCES**

Ahmann, S. J., and Glock, M. D.: Evaluating pupil growth, ed. 4, Boston, 1971, Allyn and Bacon.
Block, J. H., editor: Mastery learning, theory, and practice, New York, 1971, Holt, Rinehart & Winston, Inc.
Bloom, B. S.: Stability and change in human characteristics, New York, 1964, John Wiley & Sons, Inc.
Bloom, B. S.: Human characteristics and school learning, New York, 1976, McGraw-Hill Book Co., Inc.

Bloom, B. S.: Learning for mastery, Evaluation Comment, vol. 1, no. 2, 1968, Center for the Study of Evaluation of Instructional Programs, UCLA.

Bloom, B. S., Hastings, J. T., and Madaus, G. S.: Handbook of formative and summative evaluation of student learning, New York, 1971, McGraw-Hill Book Co., Inc.

Carroll, J. B.: A model of school learning, Teachers College Record 64(8):723-733, 1963.

Chase, C. I.: Measurement for educational evaluation, Reading, Mass., 1974, Addison-Wesley Publishing Co.

Ebel, R. L.: Essentials for educational measurement, Englewood Cliffs, N. J., 1972, Prentice-Hall, Inc.

Erickson, R. C., and Wentling, T. L.: Measuring student growth, Boston, 1976, Allyn and Bacon.

Hoyt, D. P., and Munday, L.: Academic description and prediction in junior colleges, American College Testing Program Research Reports, no. 10, Iowa City, 1966, American College Testing Program.

Husen, T., editor: International study of educational achievement in mathematics; a comparison of twelve countries, New York, 1967, John Wiley & Sons, Inc.

Mann, W. C.: Reliability of evaluative interviews for admission into health professional training (unpublished dissertation, State University of New York at Buffalo, 1977).

Martin, J. A.: Mastery learning; a model for allied health, Journal of Allied Health 6(3): 40-44, Summer 1977.

Morrison, H. C.: The practice of teaching in the secondary school, Chicago, 1932, University of Chicago Press.

Skinner, B. F.: How to teach animals, Scientific American **185**:26-29, 1951.

Skinner, B. F.: The science of learning and the art of teaching, Harvard Educational Review **24**:86-97, 1954.

Suslow, S.: Grade inflation; end of a trend? Change 9(3):44-45, March 1977.

Thorndike, R. L., and Hagen, E.: Measurement and evaluation in psychology and education, ed. 3, New York, 1969, John Wiley & Sons, Inc.

Trow, M.: Aspects of American higher education, 1969-1975, Berkeley, Calif., 1977, Carnegie Council of Policy Studies in Higher Education.

Washburne, C. W.: Educational measurements as a key to individualizing instruction and promotions, Journal of Educational Research **5**:195-206, 1922.

# Index

## A

Academic failure, noneducational causes of, 165-166
Achievement, grading based on, 166-167
Achievement tests, classroom, constructing of, 27-43
  defining objectives, 27-28
  table of specifications, 28-33
  writing directions, 33-34
  writing items, 34-42
Affective objectives, 4, 23
Anxiety, test, 147-150
  reduction of, 148-150
Auto-tutorial instruction, 20

## B

Behavior therapy and group counseling, reduction of test anxiety through, 149-150
Behavioral objectives, 4-5
Brennan's Index, 138-139

## C

Central tendency, 83-91
  mean, 88-91
  median, 86-88
  mode, 83-85
Coefficient, correlation, 60-64, 115-117
Cognitive objectives, 4, 23
Cognitive restructuring, reduction of test anxiety through, 148
Comparison questions, 14
Competency-based objectives, 3-5
Computer-assisted instruction, 21-22
Concurrent validity of tests, 59

Conference, 16
Construct validity of tests, 64-66
Content validity of tests, 59
Coping model, reduction of test anxiety through, 149
Correlation, 114-119
  interpreting, 117-118
  multiple, 118-119
  scattergrams, 115
Correlation coefficients, 60-64, 115-117
Counseling, group, and behavior therapy, reduction of test anxiety through, 149-150
Cox-Vargas Difference Index, 136-137
Criterion-related validity of tests, 59-64
Curve, normal, 97-98

## D

Deductive questions, 14
Degree of freedom (df), 120
Demonstration, 19
Descriptive questions, 13
Desensitization, self-controlled systematic, reduction of test anxiety through, 148-149
Difficulty index, 126-127
Discrimination index, 127-129
  Brennan's, 138-139
  Cox-Vargas, 136-137
Discussion
  group, 16-18
  lecture and, 11-16
Distributions
  frequency; see Frequency distributions
  skewed, 98-99
Divergent questions, 14

**E**

Equivalence reliability of tests, 67, 69-70
Error of measurement, standard, 108-109
Essay questions, 44-57
    design, 46-51
        analysis, 46-48
        evaluation, 49-51
        synthesis, 48-49
    guidelines
        for grading, 54-56
        for writing, 51-53
    types, 53-54

**F**

Factual questions, 13
Formula, Spearman-Brown Prophecy, 70
Frequency distributions, 74-83
    frequency polygon, 80, 81-83
    grouped, 76-80
        percentiles and percentile ranks for, 112-113
    histograms, 80-81
    simple, 74-76
        percentiles and percentile ranks for, 111-112
Frequency polygon, 80, 81-83

**G**

Goal statements, 3-5
Grading, 152-171
    criterion-referenced, 156-165
        advantages and limitations, 163-165
        mastery learning and, 156-163
    grade inflation, 168-169
    growth versus achievement, 166-167
    noneducational causes of academic failure, 165-166
    norm-referenced, 152-156
        advantages and limitations, 155-156
        functions, 153-155
    weighing assessment data, 167-168
Group counseling and behavior therapy, reduction of test anxiety through, 149-150
Group discussion, 16-18
Growth, grading based on, 166-167

**H**

Higher-order questions, 13-14
Histograms, 80-81

**I**

Independent study, 20
Indices, statistical, 126-129
    difficulty, 126-127
    discrimination, 127-129, 136-139
Individualized instruction, 20-22
    auto-tutorial, 20
    computer-assisted, 21-22
    programmed, 21
Inductive questions, 14
Inferences, 14
Internal consistency of tests, 67, 70-71
Item analysis; *see* Tests, item analysis of

**K**

Kuder-Richardson procedure, 70-71

**L**

Learning
    mastery, 156-163
        aptitude and, 159-160
        instruction
            ability to understand, 160-161
            quality, 160
        perseverance and, 159
        time allowed, 158-159
    strategies, 7-23
        methods, 7-22
            demonstration, 19
            group discussion, 16-18
            independent study, 20
            individualized instruction, 20-22
            laboratory method, 19
            lecture, 10-11
            lecture-discussion, 11-16
            role playing, 18-19
Lecture, 10-11
Lecture-discussion, 11-16
    questioning skills, 12-14
    reinforcement, 15-16
    set induction, 11-12
Level of significance, 120, 121

**M**

Mastery learning, 156-163
    aptitude, 159-160
    instruction
        ability to understand, 160-161
        quality, 160

Mastery learning—cont'd
  instruction—cont'd
    perseverance and, 159
    time allowed, 158-159
Matching items, writing of, for tests, 41-42
Mean, 88-91
Measurement, standard error of, 108-109
Media for instruction, 22-23
Median, 86-88
Mode, 83-85
Multiple-choice test items, writing of, 37-41

**N**

Nomological net theory, 65
Normal curve, 97-98
Nursing Board Examination scores, 106-108

**O**

Objectives
  behavioral, 4-5
  competency-based, 3-5
  instructional, and achievement testing, 27-28
  teaching method and, 7-8

**P**

Percentile band, 114
Percentiles and percentile rank, 109-114
  advantage, 114
  disadvantages, 113-114
  for grouped frequency distribution, 112-113
  percentile band, 114
  for simple frequency distribution, 111-112
Polygon, frequency, 80, 81-83
Positive reinforcement, 15-16
Practicality of tests, 71-72
Predictive validity of tests, 60
Programmed instruction, 21
Psychomotor objectives, 4, 23
Psychomotor skills, demonstration teaching of, 19
Psychosocial concerns for testing, 140-151; *see also* Testing, psychosocial concerns for

**Q**

Questioning skills, 12-14
Questions, essay, 44-57
  design, 46-51
    analysis, 46-48
    evaluation, 49-51
    synthesis, 48-49
  guidelines
    for grading, 54-56
    for writing, 51-53
  types, 53-54

**R**

Range, 91-93
Rationale statement, 2-3
Reinforcement, 15-16
Reliability of tests, 66-71
  equivalence, 67, 69-70
  internal consistency, 67, 70-71
  stability, 67-69
Role playing, 18-19

**S**

Scattergrams, 115
Scores, standard, 100-108; *see also* Standard scores
Scoring, unreliability of, in essay questions, 45-46
Set induction, 11-12
Sixteen Personality Factor Questionnaire, 72
Skewed distributions, 98-99
Spearman-Brown Prophecy Formula, 70
Stability reliability of tests, 67-69
Standard deviation, 94-96
Standard error of measurement, 108-109
Standard scores, 100-108
  Nursing Board Examination scores, 106-108
  $T$-score, 103-106
  $z$-scores, 100-103
Statistical indices, 126-129
  difficulty, 126-127
  discrimination, 127-129
Statistics, descriptive, 83-123
  central tendency, 83-91
  correlation, 114-119
  normal curve, 97-98
  percentiles and percentile ranks, 109-114

Statistics, descriptive—cont'd
skewed distributions, 98-99
standard error of measurement, 108-109
standard scores, 100-108
*t*-test, 119-122
variability, 91-97
Supply-type test items, writing of, 34-35
Systematic instructional design, 1-26
goals and objectives, 3-5
instructional revision, 24-25
learning strategies, 7-23
postassessment, 23-24
preassessment, 5-7
rationale, 2-3
Systems model for instruction, 2

**T**

Testing, psychosocial concerns for, 140-151
behaviorist approach, 140-147
extinction, 141-142
negative reinforcement, 141
positive reinforcement, 141
use of, 143-147
punishment, 142-143
test anxiety, 147-150
reduction of, 148-150
Tests
achievement; *see* Achievement tests, classroom, constructing of
item analysis of, 125-139
computer output for, 131-133
for criterion-referenced tests, 135-139
interpreting indices, 126-129

Tests—cont'd
item analysis of—cont'd
item file, 133-134
limitations, 135
manual, 129-131
purposes, 125-126
practicality, 71-72
reliability, 66-71
equivalence, 67, 69-70
internal consistency, 67, 70-71
stability, 67-69
validity, 58-66
construct, 64-66
content, 59
criterion-related, 59-64
True/false test items, writing of, 35-37
*T*-score, 103-106
*t*-Test, 119-122
for dependent means, 121-122
for independent means, 119, 120-121
interpretation, 122

**V**

Validity of tests, 58-66
construct, 64-66
content, 59
criterion-related, 59-64
Variability, 91-97
range, 91-93
standard deviation, 94-96
variance, 93-94
Variance, 93-94

**Z**

*z*-Score, 100-103